DOCTOR'S
Little Black Bag
of Remedies
& Cures

Volume 2

Table of Contents

5. MIND POWER

1. Healing Foods

FOOD AND MOOD

Folk wisdom has long held that our moods are influenced by the food we eat. That belief is gaining support from scientific research.

Food-mood strategies* can't cure clinical depression or other serious psychological disorders. These problems call for professional help. But they can be used to boost alertness at work...increase your sense of relaxation at home...and make it easier for you to tolerate life's ups and downs.

Mood-altering foods aren't unusual or hard to find. You don't have to follow a long, complex regimen before seeing results. They are ordinary, everyday foods...and in some cases, their effects are felt within as little as 30 minutes.

How food acts on our moods...

Recent research suggests that food affects mood by altering the brain's production of chemical messengers called *neurotransmitters*.

The neurotransmitters *dopamine* and *norepinephrine* have an energizing effect. When your brain is producing these chemicals, you're alert, highly motivated and have fast reaction times.

*Don't confuse food-mood effects with food allergies. True food allergies are usually accompanied by a rash, stomachache or other physical symptoms. In the absence of such symptoms, anxiety or depression is unlikely to be related to food allergy—despite the claims of many "experts." If you have symptoms of food allergy, see an allergist. Do not attempt to treat the condition yourself.

The main building block of these "alertness chemicals" is the amino acid *tyrosine*. Eating protein—which contains lots of tyrosine—raises tyrosine levels in the brain. This, in turn, boosts synthesis of dopamine and norepinephrine. *Result:* Greater mental energy.

The neurotransmitter *serotonin* has a calming effect. Its presence in the brain boosts concentration, relieves feelings of anxiety and—at night or if you're sleep-deprived—makes you feel drowsy.

To make serotonin, your brain needs a supply of the amino acid *tryptophan*. Like tyrosine, tryptophan is found in proteins. But eating more protein *won't* increase levels of tryptophan inside your brain. In fact, a high-protein diet *depletes* the brain's tryptophan supply.

Reason: Tryptophan must "compete" with tyrosine and other, more plentiful amino acids to enter the brain. It tends to be "crowded out" by them when you eat protein.

To increase the brain's supply of tryptophan, eat carbohydrates —*without protein*. Doing so triggers the release of insulin, which shunts some of the amino acids from the blood to other organs. Tryptophan, however, is left behind in the blood. With less competition from other amino acids, it can easily enter the brain.

Basic food-mood prescription...

Because tyrosine and tryptophan can be dangerous when taken in pill form, it's best to use *food* to affect levels of these neurotransmitters.

Caution: The following principles are no substitute for eating a healthful, well-balanced diet. If you have diabetes, hypoglycemia or another diet-related condition, consult a doctor before changing your eating habits.

•**For greater alertness, motivation and mental energy...eat protein.** Just three to four ounces (less than half the size of a typical restaurant entrée) is enough to get tyrosine to the brain so it can be used to make dopamine and norepinephrine.

Best sources of protein: Fish, shellfish, skinless chicken, veal, lean beef and egg whites. Because these foods are essentially pure protein—with little or no fat or carbohydrates—they work especially quickly.

Other good sources: Low-fat dairy products, dried legumes, tofu and other soy products. These contain carbohydrates but are low in fat.

Avoid: Fatty foods, such as pork, lamb, fatty cuts of beef, most hard cheeses and other whole-milk products. High-fat foods divert blood from the brain to the digestive tract. They take a very long time to digest.

•**To calm down, relax and focus...eat carbohydrates.** As little as one to one-and-one-half ounces is all most people need. Overweight people and women during the two or three days just prior to menstruation may need up to two-and-one-half ounces.

2

Eating the carbohydrate *without protein* is crucial. *Reason:* Protein will boost levels of amino acids that compete with tyrosine for entry to the brain. Instead of feeling calmer, you'll feel hyped-up. (If alertness is your goal, eating carbohydrates along with protein usually does not interfere with tyrosine's energizing effect.)

Best sources of carbohydrates: Gumdrops, licorice, marshmallows, jam and other sweets...grain-based foods such as bread, crackers, pasta, rice, popcorn and pretzels...and starchy vegetables such as potatoes.

Fruits and nonstarchy vegetables are *not* good materials for the brain's serotonin factory. A healthful diet includes plenty of both, but these are not the foods to eat when you need to feel calm or focused.

Food-mood strategies and weight-loss diets...

Dieters often wonder whether these food-mood strategies lead to overeating—and to weight gain. In fact, these strategies are more likely to promote healthful eating...

Reason #1: Very small portions are needed to produce results.

Reason #2: The recommendations call for little or no fat. Not only is fat bad for you, but it also interferes with the food-mood effect.

Mealtime power...

For consistent results, use the food-mood principles to time your intake of proteins and carbohydrates...

•**Breakfast.** It should contain protein but little or no fat. *Possibilities:* An orange, eight ounces of low-fat yogurt and a low-fat bran muffin...or cranberry juice and hot cereal with skim milk.

•**Morning snack.** A snack is OK for those who find it hard to eat even a light meal first thing in the morning...and those who eat breakfast so early that they feel hungry by midmorning. It will keep these individuals from coming to lunch so hungry that they overeat and feel sluggish all afternoon. *Good choice:* A small can of grapefruit juice, two rice cakes and one slice of skim-milk mozzarella.

•**Lunch.** It should be high in protein to keep you alert...and low in fat and calories, so you won't have to expend your energy digesting a heavy meal.

Don't *begin* lunch with a carbohydrate. If you have a roll or pasta before the entrée arrives, for example, you'll be sending tryptophan to the brain. That will dull your mental edge. *Instead:* Start your meal with a salad, juice or consommé.

•**Afternoon snack.** Few people need a snack after an energy-boosting lunch—unless they're carbohydrate cravers. For reasons we don't understand, these people start to feel irritable and scattered at midday. A handful of crackers or jelly beans will help them feel calmer and more focused.

•**Dinner.** Make sure it's high in carbohydrates if you want to relax. If you need to keep your energy up for classes or volunteer work, your dinner should be high in protein.

•**Bedtime snack.** If you have trouble unwinding at bedtime, eat one-and-one-half ounces of carbohydrates 30 minutes before retiring. (That's the equivalent of five or six graham crackers.) Make sure the snack is low in fat and protein.

Warm milk at bedtime is a *bad* idea. *Reason:* Milk contains quite a bit of protein, which most people find energizing.

Stress relief...

If you feel frazzled and need to calm down, have a small carbohydrate snack. *For fastest results:* Have a cup of cocoa with melted marshmallows. You should feel better within 20 minutes.

If you need sustenance during an all-day stressful situation—waiting to hear the results of a medical test, for example—nibble high-carbohydrate, low-fat foods. Avoid full meals. Follow this strategy for no more than a day or two at a time.

Power eating at conferences...

To avoid the exhaustion that plagues many conference-goers, bring your own light breakfast—or skip breakfast altogether. Avoid heavy coffee shop meals. Easy choices include a mini-box of fruit juice plus eight ounces of yogurt, or a single-serving box of cereal with low-fat milk and a banana.

If a buffet breakfast is part of the program, skip the hot table, where the high-fat foods are clustered. Instead, stick with fruit, cereals and low-fat muffins. During the coffee break, have coffee or tea, but skip the pastries.

At lunch, don't touch your roll until after you've eaten the protein part of the meal. If the entrée is a large serving, eat only half.

Pack a carbohydrate snack (such as graham crackers or fat-free cookies) in case you need to revive yourself during mid-afternoon presentations. Have it with a cup of coffee.

At dinner, emphasize protein if you need to be "on," carbohydrates if you're ready to unwind—just as you would at home. Wind down with a few crackers or candies at bedtime.

Source: Judith J. Wurtman, PhD, research scientist, department of brain and cognitive science, Massachusetts Institute of Technology, Cambridge. She is the author of *Managing Your Mind & Mood Through Food.* HarperCollins.

FASTING CAN BE VERY GOOD FOR YOUR HEALTH...

Fasting is a potent tool for achieving optimum health. Studies from Scandinavia, Russia and Japan suggest that a *medically supervised* fast boosts immune function and helps control arthritis, asthma, anxiety and depression.

I have seen fasting bring amazing—and lasting—benefits to patients with high blood pressure, angina, psoriasis, colitis, fibroids and lupus.

Fasting boosts longevity, too. Animals fed nutritious but very low-calorie diets live two times longer than well-fed animals.

Implication: Americans eat too much fat, sugar and protein...and consume too many calories. The long-term effects of our national overindulgence are reflected in the high incidence of high blood pressure and other chronic, degenerative diseases.

What is fasting?

Fasting means abstaining from all food and drink (except water) for a specified period of time. It does *not* mean starvation.

Soon after a fast begins (48 hours for women, 72 hours for men), the body goes into *protein-sparing* mode. It conserves essential tissues (heart, lungs, etc.) while sacrificing fat, tumors, fatty deposits in blood vessels and other nonessential tissues for fuel.

If you have broth, fruit juice or another beverage during a fast, you won't go into this protein-sparing state. *Result:* Many of the benefits of fasting will be lost.

Starvation doesn't begin until about five weeks—and that's far longer than anyone should fast. My patients' fasts usually last from one to four weeks.

Caution: For a fast of three days or longer, your doctor must monitor your blood electrolytes (sodium and potassium) to ensure that you have sufficient nutritional reserves.

For a list of health-care professionals in your area who have completed a six-month program in medical fasting, contact the International Association of Hygienic Physicians, c/o Mark Huberman, 204 Stambaugh Building, Youngstown, Ohio 44503.

Why fasting works...

Recent experiments suggest that free radicals and other harmful waste products of cellular metabolism build up inside cells. In addition, we're continually exposed to harmful compounds generated outside the body, such as food additives and natural food toxins.

Result: A gradual decline in cellular function.

Fasting affords a "quiet" interlude during which the body does a kind of "internal housecleaning." Rather than take in food—and create more waste—it eliminates existing waste. And since no energy is expended toward digestion, the body can devote more energy to healing.

Fasting is not a magic bullet...

Whatever health benefits you get from a fast, you won't maintain them if you go right back to the same unhealthful habits you had before the fast.

Fasting should *not* be used for weight control. People who fast as a quick, easy way to lose pounds usually gain the weight back once the fast is over. A long-term commitment to sound dietary practices and regular exercise is needed for lasting weight loss.

Fasting *can* give you a head start on making long-term lifestyle changes. It cleans the palate, raising its sensitivity to simple flavors. Lettuce, for example, tastes sweet after a fast. Less-healthful foods like peanut butter seem heavy and salty.

Heightened sensitivity to tastes, along with the enhanced physical and mental well-being that most people feel during a fast, helps motivate you to sustain healthful habits.

Who should not fast?

Fasting can be dangerous for women who are pregnant or nursing, and for anyone with...

- •Kidney failure.

- •Hepatitis or other liver trouble.

- •AIDS or advanced cancer.

- •A personal history of life-threatening heart arrhythmia.

Fasting interferes with certain medications, too. During a fast, taking acetaminophen can damage the liver, for example, while taking an antihypertensive drug can cause a dangerous fall in blood volume.

What to expect on a fast...

Many people believe that fasting makes one feel sick, uncomfortable or continuously hungry. Not true. Headache, fatigue, weakness, confusion and other symptoms can occur, but they usually pass after the first day or two. Hunger ends *completely* after the second day. After that, most people feel great.

How long should a fast last?

For a reasonably healthy person who wants to "cleanse" his body, a one-week fast is probably appropriate.

If you're coming down with a cold or sore throat, a day or two without food—combined with bed rest and lots of water—will help rid your body of the virus.

People with hypertension, heart disease, lupus, asthma, arthritis or another chronic ailment may need to fast for three to four weeks. A doctor's care is essential.

Preparing for a fast...

Eat mostly raw fruits and vegetables for a day or two before starting your fast. Such a diet acts as an intestinal "broom."

Too much refined or starchy food before a fast dries out the stool. (Most people have one bowel movement at the start of the fast, then no more until the fast is over.)

Other important strategies...

•**Rest.** If you plan to fast for just a few days, and your job isn't stressful, it's fine to go to work. But you'll derive greater benefit if you stay quiet and relaxed—napping, reading, listening to music, etc.

•**Drink lots of water.** Have one to three quarts (four to 12 eight-ounce glasses) a day. Water helps your body flush out wastes.

•**Avoid tea and other herbs.** During a fast, they can cause liver and kidney problems.

•**Avoid extremes of heat and cold.** Steam baths, saunas, etc. can make you dehydrated. And since you'll become cold easily while fasting, you may need to dress more warmly than usual.

•**Break your fast gradually.** Eating a big meal too soon after a fast can cause indigestion and painful elimination. *Better:* Reintroduce solid food gradually over three to four days.

Source: Joel Fuhrman, MD, a family physician and fasting specialist in Belle Mead, NJ, and a staff member of Hunterdon Medical Center in Flemington, NJ. He is the author of *Fasting and Eating for Health: A Medical Doctor's Program for Conquering Disease.* St. Martin's Press.

ALL ABOUT HERBAL REMEDIES

Even if you eat right, exercise regularly and get plenty of sleep, herbal supplements can raise your health to a whole new level.

As explained here by one of the country's leading herbalists, Dr. Daniel B. Mowrey, so-called "tonic" herbs confer an impressive array of health benefits, including increased energy and stamina…heightened immunity…reduced risk of heart disease…improved liver function…reduced joint inflammation.

If you'd like to add herbal remedies to your medicine chest, start with the following eight tonic herbs.* All are available at health-food stores.

Unlike drugs, herbal preparations are not regulated by the FDA. Ask the store clerk to recommend a reputable brand.

You can take each of these herbs on a daily basis. Or you can rotate through the list, taking each herb for a few weeks at a time. The doses listed are based on capsules containing 850 mg to 900 mg of the herb.

Caution: Consult a doctor before starting any herbal regimen—especially if you have a heart ailment or another chronic illness and/or you are using prescription or over-the-counter medications. Herbal remedies can dangerously interact with certain drugs.

If you develop a rash, nausea, hives, headaches or hay fever-like symptoms while taking an herb, stop using it immediately.

Cayenne…

Cayenne is good for the cardiovascular system. A mild stimulant, the herb also helps maintain muscle tone in the stomach and intes-

Editor's note: Certain remedies are inherently unsafe. *Comfrey, borage* and *coltsfoot* can cause liver disease…*chaparral* can cause liver disease…*mahuang* can cause a rise in blood pressure that is particularly unsafe for those with heart or thyroid disease or diabetes… *yohimbé* can cause tremors, anxiety, high blood pressure and rapid heart rate.

tinal walls and enhances digestion. Cayenne is also an excellent "activator herb," amplifying the benefits of other herbs you take.

Daily dose: Two capsules. Or use ground cayenne as a spice.

Echinacea...

Echinacea fights illness on two levels. First, it boosts levels of white blood cells, B- and T-lymphocytes and phagocytes—the key components of a healthy immune system. Second, it neutralizes invading microorganisms.

German researchers have shown that echinacea stops staph, strep and fungal infections, along with a variety of viruses.

Daily dose: Two capsules. Be sure the capsules contain the whole root in powdered form, not extract.

Used intermittently, liquid extract of echinacea makes a soothing balm for sore throats. Using an eyedropper, let a few drops fall against the back of your throat.

Garlic...

This spice helps prevent heart disease by lowering cholesterol levels and blocking formation of fatty deposits in the coronary arteries. It also boosts levels of T-cells, a critical component of the immune system.

Animal and human studies have shown that garlic also relieves arthritis. It contains sulfur compounds, which are known to have significant anti-inflammatory properties.

Daily dose: Two pills. Or use a garlic clove or garlic powder in your cooking.

Gingerroot...

Gingerroot is an excellent remedy for indigestion, constipation, diarrhea and nausea (including morning sickness). There's no good explanation for why it works. But my research suggests that ginger is even more effective than Dramamine at preventing motion sickness. It is also effective against the flu.

Be sure to buy capsules made from the *whole* gingerroot—not extract.

Daily dose: For mild motion sickness, two capsules 15 minutes before you depart (and two to four more every hour or whenever symptoms return). For serious gastrointestinal upset, take six to 12 capsules an hour.

Lapacho...

A South American herb, lapacho contains *napthoquinones* (N-factors), unique compounds that have antiviral and antibiotic properties. It's effective at preventing colds, flu and bacterial and fungal infections.

Taken in capsule or tea form, lapacho soothes painful joints...and boosts energy levels. Lapacho also stimulates activity of enzymes in the liver, enhancing its ability to remove toxins from the blood.

In Brazil, lapacho is used to treat leukemia and cervical cancer, and lapacho salve is used to treat skin cancer.

Studies suggest that the herb may also be effective against breast cancer.

Make tea by simmering the purplish paper-thin inner lining of the bark in hot water for 20 minutes, then strain and let cool. Leftover tea can be refrigerated.

Daily dose: To prevent illness, four capsules or two cups of tea. To treat an infection, six capsules or one to two quarts of tea.

Milk thistle...

One of the world's most studied plants, milk thistle is very good for the liver. By stimulating protein synthesis, it boosts levels of key liver enzymes, speeding regeneration of damaged liver tissue. It also inhibits *lypoxygenase*, an enzyme that destroys liver cells.

Recent studies show that milk thistle can help reverse the effects of hepatitis and cirrhosis.

Daily dose: Two capsules.

Pygeum extract...

Derived from the bark of an African tree, pygeum has been shown to prevent—and even cure—benign enlargement of the prostate. It contains *phytosterols*, potent anti-inflammatory compounds. Pygeum also contains *triterpenoids*, compounds that have an anti-swelling effect.

Daily dose: To prevent prostate enlargement, two capsules. To shrink an enlarged prostate, four capsules.

Yerba mate...

This South American herb boosts energy and stamina without causing the jitters that caffeine can cause. Anecdotal reports suggest that yerba mate is also effective against asthma and allergies, though the mechanism is unknown.

Yerba mate is best taken as a daily tea. Pour boiling water over yerba mate leaves, let sit for 10 minutes, then strain and serve.

Daily dose: Two to four cups.

Source: Daniel B. Mowrey, PhD, president of the American Phytotherapy Research Laboratory, a nonprofit research facility in Lehi, UT. He is the author of several books on herbal medicine, including *Herbal Tonic Therapies*. Keats Publishing.

WHY I TAKE GINSENG

While I often recommend herbs for the *treatment* of specific maladies, I believe herbs can also be used to *prevent* illness. One herb that I find especially useful is ginseng.

I began taking ginseng more than 20 years ago. Back then, my goal was to increase my energy and enhance my overall wellness. In recent years, I've noticed that I never get sick. I don't even get colds. I suspect ginseng deserves at least some of the credit.

Recent studies in Europe and especially in Russia suggest that ginseng increases the body's resistance to stress and boosts immunity. The Chinese, who have been using the herb for more than 5,000 years, believe it increases energy levels.

Many convenience stores, grocery stores, drugstores and health food stores carry ginseng products. Ginseng is available in powdered, capsule or liquid form.

Good source of ginseng products: SDV Vitamins, Box 9215, Del Ray Beach, Florida 33482. 800-738-8482.

Be sure to follow label directions. Taking too much may be overstimulating—particularly when combined with high levels of caffeine.

Price varies according to the type and quality of root, how much ginseng the product contains—and how it was processed.

Ginsana, the leading product, costs $13 to $16 for 30 capsules. This preparation has been clinically tested more than any other ginseng product on the US market.

Source: Mark Blumenthal, director of the American Botanical Council, a nonprofit organization that publishes the quarterly journal *HerbalGram*, Box 201660, Austin, TX 78720.

CURATIVE CURRY?

Rats exposed to a chemical that ordinarily causes colon cancer developed far fewer tumors when they were fed a diet high in *curcumin.*That's the ingredient that gives curry its bright orange color.

The tumors that did form in the curry-eating rats were less likely to grow and spread.

Source: Bandaru S. Reddy, PhD, chief, division of nutritional carcinogenesis, American Health Foundation, Valhalla, NY.

2. Disease-Fighting Tactics

HOW TO CUT YOUR RISK OF CANCER BY 50%

If you think cancer rates have fallen in recent years, think again. Between 1973 and 1991, US cancer incidence rose 19% in men and 12% in women.

Cancer strikes roughly two of every five Americans—and kills more than 500,000 Americans a year. These numbers are especially tragic, because *most cases of cancer are avoidable.*

We all know how important it is to avoid smoking…wear sunscreen…and drink moderately, if at all. But these are just three of *many* anti-cancer strategies. Other vital precautions…

Eat much less fat…

A high-fat diet has been linked to cancer of the colon, breast, prostate, ovary, uterus and skin. But casual attempts to limit your fat intake aren't enough.

To *really* reduce your risk, bring your fat intake to no more than 20% of total calories (instead of the 35% to 40% that's typical of most Americans). Get into the habit of choosing low-fat or nonfat salad dressings, sauces and spreads. Give up high-fat dishes. If you must eat chips, cookies, etc., look for nonfat versions.

Eat more fiber…

Dietary fiber—the component of fruits, vegetables and grains that passes undigested through the body—helps prevent colorectal and other gastrointestinal tract cancers.

Other studies suggest that fiber may lower the risk of breast cancer as well.

Aim for 25 grams of fiber a day. Start each day with a breakfast cereal that has eight to nine grams of fiber per serving. *Other fiber-rich foods:* Whole-grain bread (4 g a slice)...pear (4 g)...mango (3.7 g) ...black beans (15 g a cup).

Eat more fruits and vegetables...

Individuals who eat five to nine servings of plant foods a day have *half* the cancer risk of those who eat few fruits and vegetables. (One serving equals one-half cup of cooked vegetables, or a medium-sized apple, orange or banana.)

In addition to being full of fiber, fruits and vegetables contain potent anti-cancer compounds.

The best-known of these compounds are vitamins C and E and beta-carotene. These *antioxidants* protect the body against free radicals, unstable molecules that turn normal cells cancerous.

Fruits and vegetables also contain a family of anti-cancer compounds called *phytochemicals.* Chief among these are *sulforaphane* (found in broccoli, cabbage and other cruciferous vegetables) and *allyl sulfides* (found in garlic and onion).

Important: Vitamin supplements do not contain these vital cancer fighters.

Avoid pesticide residues...

Although pesticides pose a lesser threat than cigarette smoke and other carcinogens, they are believed to be responsible for 20,000 cases of cancer a year.

Self-defense: Carefully wash all fruits and vegetables with warm, soapy water. Buy organic produce whenever possible.

Be physically active...

There's growing evidence that exercise helps prevent cancer. A recent Harvard study showed that physically active individuals have only 30% to 80% the usual risk of colorectal cancer.

Incorporate physical activity in all aspects of your life. Take stairs instead of elevators...walk to the supermarket...bike to work.

It's also good to participate in formal exercise, such as jogging, biking, etc. *Ideal:* Thirty minutes at a time, four times a week.

Stay slim...

A recent *New England Journal of Medicine* study confirms what doctors had long suspected—that even *moderate* weight gain increases the risk of endometrial cancer and breast cancer...and possibly colon cancer.

Self-defense: Eat healthfully and get regular exercise...and consult a dietician or weight-control specialist if you find yourself getting fat.

Practice safe sex...

While cancer isn't transmitted sexually, some sexually transmitted diseases are associated with an increased risk of cancer.

To avoid nasty germs, limit your number of sex partners. Always use a latex condom unless you are certain that both you *and* your partner are disease-free and monogamous.

Reduce psychological stress...

While there is no *direct* evidence that stress causes cancer, it's prudent to include stress-reduction techniques as part of your cancer-prevention program.

Excessive stress impairs immune function, thereby permitting cancer cells to survive...and leads people to adopt unsafe health practices.

One of the easiest and most powerful stress-reduction techniques is *creative visualization.*

What to do: Sit comfortably in a quiet, dimly lit room. Close your eyes. Take three deep breaths. Tense and release your muscles from head to toe. Envision yourself in a mountain meadow, a lush valley or another soothing landscape. Don't just *see* yourself there. Try to conjure up sounds, odors, etc.

Have regular screening tests...

Successful treatment for cancer depends on early diagnosis... and the best way to catch cancer in its earliest stages is via regular screening exams. Here are the most important ones...

•**Breast cancer.** Women should perform a self-examination of their breasts once every month, with a doctor-performed exam at least once a year. *Over 50:* Have a yearly mammogram.

•**Cervical cancer.** Women should have an annual Pap smear and pelvic exam.

•**Testicular cancer.** Men should check their testicles monthly. A doctor can show you how.

•**Prostate cancer.** Men over 50 should have a digital rectal exam (DRE) and a prostate specific antigen (PSA) test annually.

•**Skin cancer.** Men and women over 40 should have an annual full-body skin examination, performed by a doctor.

•**Colorectal cancer.** Men and women over 50 should have an annual DRE and an annual blood-in-stool test, with a sigmoidoscopy (an examination of the lower bowel) every three years.

Know your family tree...

An individual's susceptibility to many forms of cancer appears to be at least partially hereditary.

You cannot change your genes, but if cancer runs in your family, you can design a personal prevention program that involves more intensive screening.

If your father developed colon cancer at 47, for example, you might get your first sigmoidoscopy in your late 30s.

Helpful: Chart your family tree, including grandparents, parents, aunts, uncles and first cousins. Indicate which relatives developed cancer, and at what age. Discuss this chart with your doctor, and work out a screening schedule that's right for you.

The question of aspirin...

Recently, a large, well-designed study found that a single aspirin taken every other day reduces the incidence of colorectal cancer by 50%. If colon cancer runs in your family, ask your doctor whether aspirin therapy makes sense for you.

Source: Moshe Shike, MD, director of clinical nutrition at Memorial Sloan-Kettering Cancer Center, and professor of medicine at Cornell University Medical Center, both in New York City. He is coauthor of *Cancer Free: The Comprehensive Cancer Prevention Program.* Simon & Schuster.

HELP FOR CANCER PATIENTS

Cancer patients who participate in group therapy experience less depression and anxiety and fewer physical complaints.

Most effective: Social support groups, in which participants express their emotions and offer mutual support. These groups provide greater benefits than *cognitive-behavioral* groups, in which participants learn ways to ease psychological stress and change depressive thought patterns.

Theory: The opportunity to air one's feelings and receive encouragement from others may do more to relieve feelings of isolation and anxiety than trying to change one's behavior.

For more information on cancer support groups in your area, contact the American Cancer Society, 800-227-2345.

Source: Ron L. Evans, MSW, a social worker at the VA Puget Sound Health Care System, Seattle. His eight-month study of 78 cancer patients was published in *Public Health Reports,* Room 1875, JFK Federal Building, Boston 02203.

EXERCISE VS. BREAST CANCER

Women who averaged four or more hours of exercise a week had a 58% lower risk of breast cancer than non-exercisers. Exercising one to three hours a week cut the risk by 20% to 30%.

Theory: Exercise alters levels of hormones that play major roles in the development of breast cancer.

Source: Leslie Bernstein, MD, professor of preventive medicine, University of Southern California, Los Angeles.

ALL ABOUT HOMEOPATHY

Homeopathy has been in use for more than 200 years, but only now is this "like-cures-like" system of healing beginning to catch on with American consumers.

More than 2.5 million Americans used homeopathic remedies in 1990. Sales of homeopathic remedies are now growing at an estimated rate of 25% a year. And yet mainstream doctors remain very skeptical of homeopathy.

What's going on? Do American consumers know something that most doctors don't? Or are homeopathic remedies a waste of money?

For the answers to these and other common questions about homeopathy, we spoke with Dr. Michael Carlston, a family physician who teaches homeopathy at the University of California–San Francisco School of Medicine...

•**What is homeopathy?** It's a system of medicine whose aim is to stimulate the body to heal itself. *Theory:* Natural substances that cause certain symptoms will cure those symptoms when given in minuscule doses.

•**Does it work?** Mainstream doctors tend to be very skeptical. I myself approached homeopathy as a skeptic. But I have watched in astonishment as homeopathic remedies helped patients whose symptoms could not be helped by orthodox medicine. In many cases, I have seen fundamental changes in the health of these individuals.

Homeopathy is especially effective against chronic conditions, including asthma, ear infections, depression, allergies and migraines. Conventional medications used to treat these conditions often have significant adverse effects. Moreover, conventional drugs only treat the *symptoms*—they don't solve the problem. Homeopathic remedies are much less likely to have adverse effects.

I've found homeopathy to be good for treating certain acute conditions as well, including diarrhea and croup.

•**Are there certain conditions for which homeopathy is ineffective?** Conditions *unlikely* to respond well to homeopathy include Alzheimer's disease, cirrhosis, glaucoma, chronic schizophrenia, cancer, cataracts, diabetes, epilepsy and Parkinson's disease.

•**What are homeopathic remedies made of?** These remedies— of which there are hundreds—are made of plants, minerals, animals or even synthetic chemicals. They are typically sold in pill form, although drops and ointments are also available.

Example: Rhus tox—a remedy used to treat poison ivy and other skin ailments—is made by soaking a poison ivy plant in alcohol, repeatedly diluting the mixture with alcohol and then dripping the solution onto sugar tablets for easy administration.

A remedy's potency is determined by the extent to which it is diluted. Paradoxically, the more dilute the remedy, the greater its potency. Potencies are designated using the letters "c" or "x." "C" remedies are more dilute—and thus more potent.

Example: A homeopathic remedy designated 1c is 100 times more potent than one designated 1x.

In general, homeopathic doctors use high potencies to treat chronic conditions and low potencies to treat acute conditions.

Example: A 30c remedy may be appropriate for a sudden attack of diarrhea. For a long-term gastrointestinal complaint, however, a 200c remedy is probably more appropriate.

•**Are the remedies safe?** Homeopathic remedies are monitored for safety by the FDA. Perhaps more reassuring, few serious problems have been attributed to them in more than 190 years of use.

I believe that homeopathic remedies are as safe and probably safer than any other over-the-counter medication—as long as they are used as directed.

One possible danger: Repeated doses of one remedy may eventually cause the very symptoms the remedy is intended to cure. For example, many parents find chamomilla effective against colic. But by continuing to give a child chamomilla even *after* the colic has disappeared, parents may bring on the very crankiness they were trying to cure in the first place.

•**How does homeopathy work?** No one really knows. Most remedies are so dilute that no trace of the original substance remains. That makes it hard, indeed, to understand how they could be effective.

Yet while its mechanism of action is still to be explained, homeopathy does work if the right remedy is prescribed. I know that from my clinical experience.

Key: Choosing the proper remedy. In orthodox medicine, any one of several drugs will have the same basic effect. In homeopathy, only *one* remedy is truly effective...and there may be 100 or more remedies to choose from for any given condition.

To find this uniquely effective remedy, I question my patients *very* closely. In treating a patient with a stubborn cold, for instance, I note the quality of the mucus...the time of day its symptoms are most severe...where the congestion is...whether it is better or worse in open air...how it is affected by hot drinks, etc. Only after I have considered all these aspects of the illness am I able to pick the proper remedy.

•**Does research support the use of homeopathy?** In a 1991 study published in the *British Medical Journal*, researchers analyzed 107 clinical trials on homeopathy. *Conclusion:* Homeopathy was most beneficial for allergies, childbirth, migraines, injuries, arthritis and influenza. The authors concluded that there was sufficient evidence to justify further research into homeopathy. They fell short of actually endorsing homeopathy—primarily because they could not explain how it worked.

Additional studies published in *The Lancet* and the *British Journal of Clinical Pharmacology* demonstrated the effectiveness of homeopathic remedies against hay fever and rheumatoid arthritis.

A 1994 study published in *Pediatrics* credited homeopathic remedies with a 20% reduction in the duration of infant diarrhea. Additional studies are under way to test homeopathy's effectiveness in treating other conditions.

•**Where can I get homeopathic remedies?** Most health food stores carry them, as do many drugstores and some supermarkets. Both *single* and *combination* remedies are available. Colds, flu and other acute illnesses respond well to self-treatment.

Ninety-five percent of homeopathic remedies are sold over the counter—no prescription necessary. The remaining 5% are rarely used but can be prescribed by anyone who meets legal prescribing criteria (see below).

•**How do I know what to buy?** Combination remedies are best for acute conditions such as flu, colds, muscle strain, insect bites, headaches and sunburn.

Having two or more remedies in a single pill makes it more likely you'll get the one remedy you need—*but doesn't guarantee it*. Different manufacturers use different formulations, so one may work better for you than another.

Though more difficult to select, single remedies are often more effective. *Reason:* They are specifically tailored to a particular pattern of symptoms. And—you can get higher potencies with single-ingredient remedies.

A single-ingredient remedy can be good for treating several different problems.

Example: Sulfur is effective against depression, asthma, sinus infection, diarrhea (acute and chronic), insomnia and certain skin conditions, including eczema and pruritus (itching).

A potency of 30c is a good bet for most conditions. Consult a homeopath before using higher potencies.

Books on homeopathic first-aid are a good source of information on treating minor conditions. For chronic conditions, however, it's better to consult a homeopathic practitioner. Homeopathy is practiced by a variety of health care professionals including medical doctors, osteopaths (DO), naturopaths (ND), dentists and chiropractors (DC).

•**How do I take the remedies?** Follow the instructions printed on the package. You can't simply gulp down the pills. First, you must have a clean mouth without the taste of food or toothpaste. Let the remedy dissolve on or under your tongue, then wait at least 10 minutes before having anything to eat or drink. Store remedies away from heat.

How quickly you respond depends largely upon how long you've had the illness. *Example:* Canker sores that developed over a period of days or weeks may take days to respond…while a teething child will often feel better within 30 minutes. The more severe the problem, the more frequently you should take the remedy.

Remedies for specific ailments…

Here are 14 common maladies and the single homeopathic remedies I use to treat them. I usually prescribe 30c potencies.

- **Canker sores.** *Mercurius vivus*…take two to five pills three times a day.
- **Croup.** When patient is coughing and fearful, *aconite*…two to five pills hourly for two hours, then up to every few hours as needed. If the patient is irritable rather than fearful, try *hepar sulph*.
- **Cuts and abrasions.** *Calendula* ointment.
- **Grief or sadness.** *Ignatia amara* once daily for one to two weeks.
- **Hemorrhoids.** Homeopathic salves with *aesculus, hamamelis* and *collinsonia*. Apply after each bowel movement.
- **Insect bites or punctures with redness or swelling.** *Ledum* …two to five pills every four hours.
- **Minor injuries with bruising.** *Arnica montana*…two to five pills. Frequency depends on injury severity. For pain due to fracture, take every 15 minutes. For muscle strain, take three times a day.
- **Menstrual cramps.** *Magnesia phosphorica*…two to five pills every two to four hours as needed.
- **Motion sickness.** *Cocculus* for dizziness, *tabacum* for nausea… two to five pills every two hours as needed.
- **Panic attack or emotional shock.** *Aconite*…two to five pills as often as every 10 minutes.
- **Rashes.** For contact dermatitis and other itchy rashes that are worsened by heat, *sulfur*. For poison ivy, when the itching is relieved from a hot shower or bath, *rhus tox*. For hives, *apis*. Take two to five pills as often as needed.
- **Stage fright.** *Gelsemium*…two to five pills.
- **Teething.** *Chamomilla*…two to five pills every four hours as needed.
- **Vomiting with diarrhea.** *Veratrum album*…two pills up to every few hours as needed. *Also helpful: Arsenicum album* and *phosphorus*.

Source: Michael Carlston, MD, a board-certified family practitioner in Santa Rosa, CA, and an assistant clinical professor of family and community medicine at the University of California–San Francisco School of Medicine.

GREEN TEA VS. HEART DISEASE

Green tea may help prevent heart disease as well as cancer. It apparently does so by lowering total cholesterol and raising levels of high-density-lipoprotein (good) cholesterol. And—recent research suggests that green tea may also help protect against liver disorders.

Source: Kazue Imai, LittD, department of epidemiology, Saitama Cancer Center Research Institute, Saitami, Japan. Her study of green tea consumption in 1,371 men age 40 or older was published in the *British Medical Journal*, Tavistock Square, London WCIH 9JR, England.

WARMING THE HEART

Warm baths may be good for patients with *congestive heart failure* (enlarged heart). But check with your doctor first.

Previously, hot baths were thought to stress the heart. But in a recent study, patients who spent 15 minutes in a 106°F bath or a 140°F sauna experienced increased cardiac output and improved pumping efficiency. *Theory:* Body warmth boosts blood flow to the heart and lungs.

Source: Chuwa Tei, MD, senior research scientist, Mayo Clinic, Rochester, MN.

HEALING MAGNETS

In China, France, Japan and especially in India, magnetic therapy has long been used to speed the healing of broken bones and soft-tissue injuries.

In the US, magnetic therapy is sometimes considered a form of quackery. But following the publication of several "pro-magnet" studies in the *Journal of Electro- and Magnetobiology* and other prestigious American medical journals, a few pioneering doctors in this country are starting to use magnets in their practices.

Already, magnetic therapy has proven effective at treating slow-healing fractures and arthritic knees and necks. Studies also suggest that regular use of magnets may reverse osteoporosis...prevent heart disease...slow tumor growth...and boost mental function in Alzheimer's patients.

I know from personal experience that people sleep better and wake up feeling more refreshed after a night on a magnetic mattress. I sleep on one myself!

Is magnetic therapy safe? *Absolutely.* Magnetic resonance imaging (MRI) machines routinely expose patients to magnetic fields as high as 15,000 gauss—with no negative effects. It stands to reason that a medical magnet rated at 200 to 800 gauss poses little threat.

How magnets work...

Recent studies have demonstrated quite clearly that when placed directly on the skin, a simple, handheld magnet...

•**Increases blood flow.** It does so by stimulating cellular activity through the so-called "Hall effect." This is general heating of the magnetized area.

Some scientists think magnets improve the functioning of the autonomic nervous system, which could also stimulate blood flow to the affected area.

•**Diminishes pain.** This occurs via a combination of the Hall effect and possibly some stabilizing influence on the autonomic nervous system.

•**Speeds healing.** It does so by boosting the body's synthesis of *adenosine triphosphate* (ATP), the "fuel" that fires all cellular processes...and by enhancing the blood's ability to carry oxygen.

Magnets versus arthritis...

Magnetic therapy helps relieve arthritis pain *and* slows the deterioration of cartilage inside arthritic joints.

For my patients with arthritis, I recommend sleeping on a magnetic mattress pad...or wrapping a flexible, magnetic bandage around the affected joint. If you do sleep on a magnetic pad, remove it for a day or two, every two to four weeks. This seems to prolong the beneficial effects.

Headaches and back pain...

Magnetic pillow liners appear to be an effective treatment for chronic headaches and jaw pain.

People with chronic back pain have obtained significant relief from sleeping on magnetic mattresses, and/or using magnetic seat cushions.

Soft tissue inflammation...

Tennis elbow, carpal tunnel syndrome and other tendon or ligament problems heal faster when wrapped in magnetic bandages.

In most cases, the magnet is wrapped into place over the affected area—and left in place until the pain disappears.

Broken bones...

In some hospitals, powerful electromagnets are being used to speed healing of stubborn bone fractures. Magnetic therapy also seems to promote regeneration of spinal disk tissue.

Asthma...

Regular use of magnets helps prevent the violent allergic reaction in the lungs that is characteristic of bronchial asthma.

Helpful: Sleeping on a magnetic mattress...or wearing a magnetic bandage on your chest.

Putting magnets to work...

The benefits of magnetic therapy are often apparent within the first hour of treatment. In others, three or four days of steady treatment are required.

For maximum benefit: Place magnets as close to your body as possible. The strength of the magnetic field drops off sharply with distance.

A variety of magnetic devices is now available—including mattress pads, seat cushions, pillow liners, magnet-studded bandages and simple handheld magnets.

Good source of medical magnets: Norso Biomagnetics, 4105 Starboard Ct., Raleigh, North Carolina 27613. 800-480-8601.

Source: Ron Lawrence, MD, a neurologist in private practice in Agoura Hills, CA. He is president of the newly formed North American Academy of Magnetic Therapy, 17445 Oak Creek Ct., Encino, CA 91316.

CHRONOBIOLOGY

The Biblical idea that there's "a time for every purpose under heaven" is gaining scientific support. Recent research tells us that like all living things, the human body follows an internal rhythm that mirrors the cosmic cycle, creating a day and night in every single cell.

Directed by a master clock in our brains, hundreds of bodily functions wax and wane every 24 hours, helping us live efficiently on our 24-hour planet.

There's a time when our reflexes are fastest …a time when we're most creative…a time to nap…a time to hold important meetings …a time to eat…and a time to refrain from eating.

The study of these daily rhythms* is called *chronobiology.* Here's how to put this science to work for you…

The right time…

Over the course of a day, physiological functions—alertness, physical capabilities, etc.—change in response to signals from a region of the brain called the *hypothalamus.*

Time of day makes an enormous difference. According to one researcher, the decline in cognitive ability that occurs from peak to trough is roughly equivalent to the effect of three or four alcoholic drinks—or the loss of a half night of sleep.

By taking these cyclical fluctuations into account, you can plan your day for peak performance…

•**7 a.m. to 8 a.m.** As soon as possible after you wake up, expose yourself to bright light—preferably sunlight—even if it's overcast. That will help you become alert faster.

•**9 a.m. to noon.** During this three-hour span, we reason most clearly, concentrate best and are most creative. It is an ideal time for tackling the day's most intellectually demanding tasks.

*These rhythms are unrelated to biorhythms, a pseudoscientific system that claims to identify critical days on the basis of one's birth date.

•**11 a.m.** Most people are sharp, attentive and cooperative at this time. Short-term memory is at its peak, fostering intelligent dialogue. It is a good time to schedule important meetings.

•**Noon.** Complex decision-making skills are in high gear.

•**1 p.m. to 2 p.m.** People tend to be particularly cheerful at this time of day, so it's a good time for a harmonious lunch. Food eaten now is burned more efficiently than food eaten later in the day. That's why it's best for dieters to make lunch a bigger meal than dinner.

•**2 p.m.** Daydreaming peaks. Not a good time for adding numbers, monitoring dials, performing high-vigilance tasks...but poets and novelists may find this a particularly creative hour. If you must perform high-vigilance tasks at this time, schedule frequent breaks.

•**2 p.m. to 3 p.m.** Alertness ebbs during this "after-lunch" period —whether you eat lunch or not. Because drowsiness is such a problem now, it's a poor time for meetings, driving and focused thinking.

•**3 p.m.** Early-afternoon blahs are starting to lift. This is an ideal time for sorting the mail, typing and other mundane physical tasks ...and for dental appointments. *Reason:* Your sensitivity to pain is at its lowest point, and your dentist's hand steadiest.

•**3 p.m. to 5 p.m.** Long-term memory is at its peak. A good time to take classes or commit things to memory.

•**4 p.m.** Use this time to proofread letters, review contracts, check details. Your ability to detect errors peaks from now through early evening. *Also:* Plan tomorrow's schedule.

•**5 p.m.** This is the best time of day to work out. Your coordination is peaking, as are your strength and reflexes. Workouts are more enjoyable, too.

•**5 p.m. to 7 p.m.** Taste and smell are especially acute. A good time for your evening meal.

•**8 p.m. to 10 p.m.** Alertness is still high enough to do bills, read, socialize.

Fortunately, the body's timetable can be overridden—at least to some extent. Being physically active, socializing with friends or simply being under psychological stress can fill you with energy during the early-afternoon slump.

A surge of nervous adrenaline can keep you on your toes while delivering a 3 p.m. presentation. (Just don't count on an alert, attentive audience.) Your body is most sensitive to the energizing effects of caffeine in the afternoon —when you're likely to need it most.

Sleep rhythms...

Your body clock doesn't shut down while you sleep. Every 90 minutes or so, your brain cycles between dream sleep and deeper, nondream stages. However, the most restorative portion of your slumber takes place in *the first four hours* after you retire.

If for some reason it's impossible to get a full night's sleep, go to bed at your normal time and get up early.

To fall asleep fast and stay asleep through the night, it's important to keep regular hours. That means going to bed and waking up at roughly the same time—on weekends as well as on weekdays.

If you get up in the middle of the night to use the bathroom, do *not* turn on bright lights. *Reason:* Your body is especially sensitive to light at around 4 a.m. If you turn on a bright light at this time, you're programming your body to awaken at the same time the next morning.

Better: Use a night-light to find your way around at night.

Afternoon naps are also programmed into our internal clocks. If you take a daily nap, schedule it for approximately 12 hours after the midpoint of your previous night's sleep (3 p.m., if you slept from 11 p.m. to 7 a.m.). A nap taken at that time will be more restful and restorative than a nap taken at any other time of the day.

Surprisingly, sexual pleasure and fertility do not seem to be linked to time of day. However, many men find that their erections are strongest immediately after wakening.

Natural variations...

Not all adults live on exactly the same timetable. "Larks" become alert early in the morning. "Owls" don't feel fully functional until late in the day.

Understanding these natural variations can be important—especially in families with adolescent children.

From puberty through the early 20s, the body clock runs on a late schedule. A teenager who stays up until 2 a.m. or 3 a.m. and sleeps until mid-morning is only doing what comes naturally. To reflect this reality, at least one state's medical society has adopted a resolution urging a change in the high school schedule.

Sickness and health...

Blood pressure, blood sugar, heart and respiration rate and other physiological functions vary throughout the day. Fluctuations in metabolism can render the same medication considerably more potent at 9 a.m. than at 9 p.m. (or vice versa). For this reason, timing is often crucial in the case of chemotherapy drugs and other powerful, potentially toxic medications.

Some diseases are clearly worse at certain times. Asthma attacks tend to strike in the morning, for example, and osteoarthritis is most severe in late afternoon. Your doctor should take biological rhythms into account when prescribing medication.

Few doctors have much knowledge of or interest in biological rhythms—but it may be worth trying to find one who does. Ask your doctor if biological rhythms are important in your illness. If he/she doesn't know, ask your local librarian to help you do an on-line computer search on your illness and on "biological rhythms." Then make a printout for your doctor.

Pharmaceutical manufacturers are certainly taking an interest in chronobiology. One drug company is now testing a heart drug that releases its active ingredient at different rates over the course of a day—in sync with the body's ever-changing metabolism.

What you can do now: If you're concerned about your blood pressure, have it checked at several different times of the day. An individual whose blood pressure is always normal in the morning may have high blood pressure at other times of the day.

If you have arthritis or another chronic disease, become aware of the daily cycle of your symptoms. Discuss adjusting your medication schedule with your doctor. Pay attention to your body. See if your symptoms vary during the day and if the hour you take medicine makes any difference.

Source: Lynne Lamberg, a science writer and the author of *Bodyrhythms: Biological Clocks and Peak Performance*. William Morrow.

EXERCISE VS. ALZHEIMER'S DISEASE

Exercise keeps your mind sharp as you age…and may even help prevent Alzheimer's disease. In a recent study, rats that exercised regularly had elevated levels of *brain-derived neurotrophic factor*, a natural compound that keeps brain cells healthy. Levels remained high as long as the rats continued to get regular exercise.

Implication: Frequent, intermittent exercise may be the best way to gain this protective effect.

Source: Carl W. Cotman, PhD, professor of psychobiology, University of California, Irvine.

ASTHMA RELIEF

A daily supplement containing at least 500 mg of vitamin C reduces the frequency of respiratory infections and asthma attacks …and helps control nasal congestion, watery eyes and other allergy symptoms.

Source: Leonard Bielory, MD, director, asthma and allergy research center, University of Medicine and Dentistry of New Jersey–New Jersey Medical School, Newark.

DR. ALAN GABY UNCOVERS THE HIDDEN CAUSES OF OSTEOPOROSIS

It's hard to overstate the threat posed by osteoporosis. Each year, brittle bones cause 1.3 million fractures…and 50,000 elderly people—mostly women—die as a result of broken hips caused by osteoporosis.

Many women think they can avoid osteoporosis simply by drinking milk or taking calcium supplements. In fact, calcium is only one of many essential ingredients for healthy bones.

How bone is made...

The human skeleton is a complex and constantly changing system of cells.

In a constant adding/taking away process called remodeling, *osteoclast* cells secrete acids that break down old, damaged bone... while *osteoblast* cells make *osteocalcin*, a protein that draws calcium from the blood to make new bone.

Bone remodeling can be hindered by certain foods...

•**Sugar.** The average adult eats the equivalent of 41 teaspoons of refined sugar a day. *Danger:* People who eat lots of sugar excrete lots of calcium in their urine—*including calcium leached from the skeleton.* Each calcium ion that's lost leaves the bones correspondingly weaker.

Excess sugar also boosts synthesis of *cortisol*, a hormone that seems to promote osteoporosis.

•**Caffeine.** Like sugar, it boosts calcium excretion. Heavy intake of coffee, tea, soft drinks and other caffeinated beverages has been linked to an increased risk of hip fracture.

•**Alcohol.** Heavy drinkers face an increased risk of hip fracture. Alcohol weakens bone, and heavy drinkers tend to fall down.

•**Refined grains.** White flour, white bread and other foods made of refined grains often lack vitamin B-complex, folic acid, calcium, magnesium, manganese, copper, zinc and other key nutrients.

•**Protein.** Plant protein doesn't seem to cause trouble, but excessive intake of animal protein can cause bone loss via two mechanisms...

Mechanism I: Animal protein—especially meat and fish—is rich in phosphorus. Too much of this mineral upsets the body's metabolism of minerals, promoting calcium depletion.

Mechanism II: The amino acid *methionine* (found mainly in meat and milk products) is broken down into *homocysteine*, a compound that weakens bone. People with a hereditary predisposition to high homocysteine levels get osteoporosis as early as age 20.

The anti-osteoporosis diet...

To reduce your risk of osteoporosis, limit your intake of these bone-weakening foods. Instead, eat a high-fiber, low-fat diet that stresses...

...*whole grains* like brown rice and whole-wheat bread.

...*nuts, seeds and beans.*

...*fresh fruits and vegetables.* Include lots of calcium-rich, dark-green, leafy vegetables (kale, collards, etc.). Spinach and rhubarb are rich in calcium, but they contain *oxalates*, compounds that interfere with calcium absorption.

Eat vegetables raw or lightly steamed. Overcooking depletes them of calcium.

Nutritional supplements...

To get all the vitamins and minerals needed for healthy bones, I urge my patients to take supplements* containing...

•**Calcium.** Which type of calcium is best? Calcium gluconate? Calcium carbonate? Calcium citrate? In fact, no good research exists on this matter.

Whatever form you take, stick with capsules or *chewable* tablets. They dissolve quickly and completely, delivering the entire dose of calcium. If you prefer ordinary tablets, make sure they dissolve well. *Test:* Place a tablet in six ounces of vinegar at room temperature. Stir every two minutes. Within 30 minutes, the tablet should disintegrate into fine particles. If not, find a supplement that does. *Daily dose:* 600 to 1,200 mg.

•**Vitamin B-6.** Many cases of osteoporosis stem from a B-6 deficiency. B-6 promotes breakdown of homocysteine. *Daily dose:* 25 to 50 mg.

•**Vitamin K.** The body uses vitamin K to make osteocalcin. *Daily dose:* 150 to 500 micrograms (mcg).

•**Manganese.** This mineral boosts synthesis of *mucopolysaccharides*, compounds that promote formation of calcium crystals within the bones (the calcification process). *Daily dose:* 15 to 20 mg.

•**Magnesium.** A magnesium deficiency disrupts the calcification process...and poorly formed crystals mean weak bones. A recent study found increased bone density in postmenopausal women who took a magnesium supplement. *Daily dose:* 250 to 600 mg.

•**Folic acid.** This B vitamin helps rid the body of homocysteine.

Recently, postmenopausal women given 5 mg of folic acid daily showed significant reductions in homocysteine levels.

It's unclear what dose of folic acid is optimal. The recommended daily allowance is 0.4 mg. Most multivitamins contain 0.4 to 0.8 mg. Don't take more than 1 mg a day without consulting a doctor.

•**Vitamin C.** Found in citrus fruits, potatoes and other vegetables, this vitamin boosts synthesis of structural proteins in bone. *Daily dose:* 500 mg.

•**Vitamin D.** It's essential for proper calcium absorption. Most people get enough sunshine for their skin to make adequate supplies of vitamin D. If you rarely get outside, take 200 to 400 international units (IU) of vitamin D a day.

•**Zinc.** This mineral is required for the formation of osteoblasts and osteoclasts. It also aids in calcium absorption. *Daily dose:* 15 to 30 mg of zinc picolinate, zinc citrate or chelated zinc.

*Consult your doctor before taking any supplement, especially if you take other medications.

•**Boron.** This trace mineral limits calcium excretion and slows the loss of bone-protecting hormones during menopause. *Daily dose:* 1 to 3 mg.

•**Strontium.** It imparts additional strength to calcium crystals, inhibiting resorption. *Daily dose:* 0.5 to 3 mg.

•**Copper.** Animal studies show that copper deficiency leads to reduced bone strength and mineral content. Copper seems to inhibit bone resorption. *Daily dose:* 1 to 2 mg.

•**Silicon.** It plays a key role in calcification and in collagen production. It can be taken as a supplement...or obtained from *horsetail*, an herbal remedy sold at health-food stores. The optimal dose is unknown, but 1 mg a day is reasonable.

Toxic metals weaken bones...

In recent years, scientists have found that brittle bones seem to arise, in part, from the accumulation of toxic metals in the body...

•*Aluminum* **interferes with bone remodeling.** *Self-defense:* Avoid aluminum-based antacids and antiperspirants...baking powder that contains aluminum...aluminum-containing food preservatives...pickled foods. Avoid foods and beverages sold in aluminum cans.

•*Lead* **can cause bone abnormalities.** It's found in canned foods, polluted air and soil, tap water, paint, plates and cosmetics.

Self-defense: Choose jars over cans...and use lead-free paint and cosmetics. Have your water tested. If lead is found, get a water filter or drink bottled water.

•*Cadmium* **can cause bone abnormalities.** It's found in cigarette smoke and is used in making everything from batteries to fertilizer. Cadmium is ubiquitous, so it's hard to limit your exposure. But anyone can make an effort to avoid smoke.

•*Tin* **interferes with bone remodeling.** It leaches into foods and beverages from uncoated metal cans. Tin can also be found in food preservatives and toothpaste.

Self-defense: Buy foods in glass or plastic containers...buy toothpaste with calcium fluoride or sodium fluoride instead of stannous (tin) fluoride...avoid food preservatives.

The importance of exercise...

Physical activity helps prevent osteoporosis by stimulating the remodeling process. Recent research suggests that exercise can also *reverse* bone loss.

Best: Weight-bearing exercise like walking, running, tennis and weight-lifting.

Source: Alan Gaby, MD, former advisor to the National Institutes of Health Office of Alternative Medicine, and president of the American Holistic Medical Association, 4101 Lake Boone Trail, Ste. 201, Raleigh, NC 27607. He is the author of *Preventing and Reversing Osteoporosis*. Prima Publishing.

3. Solutions to Common Problems

HOW TO AVOID THE ALL-TOO-COMMON COMMON COLD

•**What causes colds?** Colds are caused by any of several *hundred* different viruses specially adapted to grow in the nose (rhinoviruses and coronaviruses). That's why it's proven impossible—so far—to make a reliable vaccine. We simply haven't been able to come up with one that's effective against all the viruses.

Smokers are particularly vulnerable to colds. Tobacco smoke dries out the mucous membranes lining the mouth and nose, impairing their ability to fend off viruses. Moderate drinkers (those who have the equivalent of one glass of wine a day) seem to be less susceptible.

One thing that does *not* affect your risk of catching a cold is *being* cold. Over the years, there have been various studies in which volunteers got soaked in cold baths or stood out in the rain. These people did *not* catch colds at a higher rate than people who stayed warm and dry.

This doesn't mean it's a good idea to go out in wintry weather without warm clothing. Being cold *can* precipitate bacterial pneumonia and other serious ailments.

•**How do colds spread?** Scientists disagree on this. Many think the virus spreads when a person inhales tiny virus-laden droplets of mucus and saliva liberated by the sneeze of an infected person.

Some evidence suggests that it's possible to catch a cold simply by being close (within a yard or so) to an infected person.

Other scientists think the virus spreads via hand-to-hand contact ...or by touching an object recently touched by an infected person, then touching the germ-laden hand to the face.

•**What can I do to avoid colds?** Since we can't count on others to stay at home when they're ill, it pays to avoid sitting or standing near anyone you suspect has a cold...and to watch where you put your hands.

•**Does vitamin C prevent colds?** Despite its popularity, vitamin C has never been proven either to prevent or cure colds. Study after study has found no real difference in the incidence, duration or severity of colds between people who took vitamin C (up to 3,000 milligrams a day) and those who did not take C.

•**What about flu shots?** They prevent certain types of influenza but won't keep you from catching a cold.

•**Does psychological stress increase my vulnerability to colds?** Absolutely. Several years ago, I did a series of studies in collaboration with Sheldon Cohen, PhD, a Carnegie Mellon University psychologist. We found that people who had recently been through a stressful experience—job loss, the death of a close relative or even *desirable* forms of stress like getting married—were more prone to colds than other individuals.

We found an almost twofold difference in infection rates among the most- and least- stressed individuals.

•**What's the best way to treat a cold?** While there's no way to cure the common cold, there are ways to make the symptoms more bearable...

•Drink liquids to keep mucous membranes moist.

•Soothe a sore throat with warm, sweet drinks, such as tea with honey. Or gargle with salt water.

•Inhale water vapor from a steam kettle or a hot bath or shower to help clear nasal passages. A hot bath is relaxing as well.

•Keep air moist with a humidifier or a kettle.

•**What about over-the-counter medications?** Take aspirin, acetaminophen or ibuprofen to reduce pain and fever. Aspirin should not be given to children under 12 because of the risk of Reye's syndrome. Aspirin can cause stomach upset, and acetaminophen occasionally causes liver damage. Ibuprofen has a good safety record, although it, too, can cause stomach upset.

A decongestant containing *ephedrine* constricts dilated blood vessels, reducing swelling and secretion of mucus. It's best to take this drug in nose drops or nasal spray, because the effect will be localized. Taking any drug orally exposes the entire body to its effects.

Never use a decongestant for more than a week. If you do, you risk a "rebound" reaction, in which congestion worsens and the body becomes dependent on the drug.

•Should I see a doctor if I have a cold? In most cases, that's unnecessary. But if symptoms persist for more than a week, or you have high fever or a pus-like nasal secretion, you may have developed a bacterial infection on top of your cold.

In such cases, see a doctor immediately. Ask if you need antibiotics—which, by the way, are *ineffective* against colds.

Children under age three, elderly people and those with lung or heart trouble are at greater risk of potentially deadly complications. They should notify a doctor at the first sign of anything more than a very mild cold.

The doctor should also determine whether you have a cold or the flu. A mild case of flu is often indistinguishable from a cold...and a severe cold may resemble the flu. Although both are characterized by sore throat, runny nose and cough, influenza usually involves muscle aches, headache and high fever.

The antiviral drugs *rimantidine* (Flumadine) and *amantidine* (Symadine) can hasten recovery of Type A influenza. However, they're effective only if taken soon after the onset of symptoms.

•Is it okay to exercise with a cold? There's no evidence that exercise prolongs or exacerbates a cold. Indeed, some people say they feel better afterward. But don't push yourself if you feel terrible.

•Are any popular home remedies helpful? Many old-fashioned remedies do seem to reduce discomfort, even if they don't actually get rid of the cold. For example, warm liquids like chicken soup soothe the throat, while the rising steam loosens up mucus. And tea made with ginger or another fragrant herb helps settle an upset stomach.

Menthol—mixed with hot water to make steam or rubbed in gel form on the upper lip—seems to clear clogged nasal passages.

Zinc lozenges, the herb *echinacea* and homeopathic products are said to help cure colds. But scientific studies have never confirmed their effectiveness.

•What about those mechanical devices that blow hot air up the nose? There's no evidence that these hair-dryer-like devices, which were popular a few years ago, do much good. They may relieve some symptoms, but they won't make your cold go away.

You can derive the same benefit by inhaling the steam from a bowl of soup or hot water.

Source: David A. J. Tyrrell, MD, who has been studying the common cold for more than 35 years. Now a health care consultant, Dr. Tyrrell is the former director of the Common Cold Unit of the Medical Research Council in Salisbury, England.

WHY ARE YOU TIRED ALL THE TIME?

If you feel tired all the time, you have lots of company. Each year, Americans make 500 million visits to the doctor seeking treatment for fatigue.

Many people who frequently feel tired fear they have the debilitating condition *chronic fatigue and immune dysfunction syndrome* (CFIDS).

If your fatigue has persisted for more than six months or is accompanied by sleep disturbances, joint pain, headaches, inability to concentrate or short-term memory loss, you may indeed have CFIDS.

In such cases, it's best to seek treatment from a CFIDS specialist. For a list of specialists in your area, contact the CFIDS Association, Box 220398, Charlotte, North Carolina 28222. 800-442-3437.

Good news: Only about 10% of my patients with fatigue actually have CFIDS. The rest are suffering from "garden variety" fatigue, caused by too little sleep or exercise, poor dietary habits or other easily correctable problems.

Thyroid problems...

Many cases of chronic fatigue are caused by over- or underproduction of *thyroxine*. That's the thyroid hormone responsible for regulating how energy is consumed by the body's cells.

Overactive thyroid: Symptoms of *hyper*thyroidism include fatigue, anxiety, insomnia, heart palpitations and bulging eyes. This condition is treated with thyroxine-blocking drugs...or with surgery or radioactive iodine to destroy the thyroid gland.

Underactive thyroid: Suspect *hypo*thyroidism if you feel depressed or lethargic, chill easily, are gaining weight or suffer from premenstrual syndrome (PMS), muscle aches, dry skin, eczema, hair loss, low libido, a hoarse throat or frequent colds or flu.

If you're experiencing any of these symptoms, it's a good idea to check your basal body temperature. Insert a thermometer under your armpit as soon as you awaken, before getting out of bed. Record results for three consecutive mornings.

A basal temperature of 97.4 degrees or lower suggests hypothyroidism. Your doctor can give you a blood test to confirm your suspicions.

Most doctors treat hypothyroidism with synthetic thyroxine (*synthroid*). However, some patients show more improvement when they take natural thyroid hormone (derived from beef or pork).

If synthroid doesn't relieve your symptoms, ask your doctor to consider that alternative.

Adrenal insufficiency...

Anyone whose fatigue is accompanied by malaise, frequent illness, allergies or low blood pressure or sugar may be making too little of the adrenal hormone *dehydroepiandrosterone* (DHEA).

31

Adrenal insufficiency is usually caused by autoimmune disease …or by adrenal gland damage stemming from long-term use of cortisone.

If a blood test reveals low levels of DHEA, you might need to take it in pill form.

In Europe, DHEA has long been used to boost immune function and combat fatigue—though few American doctors have much experience with the drug.

To find an endocrinologist familiar with DHEA, call the American College for Advancement in Medicine (714-583-7666).

Diabetes…

Adult-onset diabetes is an often-overlooked source of persistent fatigue. To rule out this condition, ask your doctor for a *fasting blood glucose test.*

The normal range of insulin is 80 to 100 mg per deciliter of blood. If you fall above that range, eating a special diet and getting regular exercise can help lower blood sugar levels. That should boost your energy.

Hormonal problems…

In men, some cases of chronic fatigue are caused by abnormally low levels of testosterone. Men suffering from this problem (which can be spotted with a simple blood test) can boost energy levels by taking testosterone supplements.

Hormone problems can cause fatigue in women, too. But tests for hormone imbalances in women are often inaccurate.

Instead of relying on a blood test, women should suspect hormone problems if…

…their fatigue is cyclical, getting worse prior to menstruation and improving afterward.

…they experience weight gain of more than five pounds prior to each period.

…they perpetually crave sugar, spicy foods or chocolate.

…they experience migraines or breast tenderness when taking birth-control pills.

To treat hormone-related fatigue, women should reduce their consumption of alcohol, meat and dairy products…eat more dietary fiber and less sugar and refined foods…take supplements of *gamma linolenic acid* (GLA).

GLA is found in primrose oil, borage oil and black currant seed oil, available at health-food stores.

Women with extreme PMS-related fatigue should ask the doctor about having a *Meyer's cocktail* once a month. That's an intravenous drip of magnesium, calcium and vitamins C and B.

Food allergies…

Chronic, mild food allergies can cause fatigue. Suspect allergies if you have dark circles under your eyes…are frequently irritable …feel foggy or depressed…or have frequent infections or dry skin.

Cravings for particular foods or cycles of energy and fatigue also suggest food allergies—especially to wheat and dairy products. These foods can cause the body to produce an energy-sapping morphine-like substance.

Consider a medically supervised fast of one to four days, to see if your energy increases. Add foods back to your diet only with the doctor's permission.

Environmental toxins...

If you can't find another source of fatigue, you may be suffering from exposure to indoor pollutants. *Usual culprits:*

•**Formaldehyde.** In carpets and drapes.

•**Nitrogen dioxide.** Released by kerosene heaters, gas stoves and furnaces.

•**Lead.** In tap water and house paint.

•**Trichloroethylene.** Used in dry cleaning.

•**Mercury.** In dental fillings and in some house paints.

•**Benzene.** In linoleum and degreasers.

Have your home tested for environmental toxins. For companies that test air and water, look under "Laboratories–Testing"—in the Yellow Pages. One reputable firm is RCI Environmental, 17754 Preston Rd., Ste. 101, Dallas 75252. 214-250-6608.

If toxins *are* a problem, install carbon-based water and air filters. Make sure your home is well-ventilated so that fumes can escape. Fill your home with houseplants to help filter the air.

Your doctor should test your blood for chemical markers of contaminants...and your hair for lead, mercury and other toxic metals. If traces of toxins are found, ask him/her about adding selenium, vitamin E, beta-carotene, garlic and sodium alginate to your diet. They help rid the body of toxic metals.

For a free list of doctors in your area who will perform such tests, send a self-addressed, stamped envelope to the American Academy of Environmental Medicine, Box CN1001-8001, New Hope, PA 18938. 215-862-4544.

For more information on environmental toxins, contact the Human Ecology Action League, Box 29629, Atlanta 30359. 404-248-1898.

The role of sugar...

In many cases, fatigue is the result of eating too much sugar.

Sugar and refined carbohydrates make your blood sugar rise. This signals the pancreas to produce insulin. Too much insulin leads to *hypoglycemia* (low blood sugar), which causes extreme fatigue.

If you suspect hypoglycemia, ask your doctor for an *oral glucose-tolerance test.* If, during the test, you experience heart palpitations, mental confusion or extreme fatigue, or feel dizzy or shaky, suspect a sugar problem—even if your doctor says your blood sugar levels are normal.

Treatment is simple—stop eating sugar. *Also helpful:* Eating six small meals instead of the usual three big meals. Small, frequent meals help stabilize blood sugar levels.

Finally, ask your doctor about taking ergogenic (energy-generating) dietary supplements, including vitamin B-15...L-carnitine... octacosanol, a wheat germ extract...ginseng.

Source: Ronald L. Hoffman, MD, director of the Hoffman Center for Holistic Medicine in New York City and host of the syndicated daily radio program "Healthtalk." He is the author of *Tired All the Time: How to Regain Your Lost Energy.* Pocket Books.

HYPNOSIS VS. HEADACHES

Headaches during pregnancy can often be relieved via hypnosis. In a recent study, symptoms improved in 80% of women who received training in hypnosis, along with physical therapy. In some cases, the relief lasted for up to a year following childbirth.

Advantage: Since no drugs are involved, there is no risk to the fetus.

Source: Dawn Marcus, MD, assistant professor of neurology, University of Pittsburgh School of Medicine Pain Institute. Her study of 44 pregnant women with migraine, tension or other types of headaches was presented at a meeting of the American Pain Society, 5700 Old Orchard Rd., Skokie, IL 60077.

WATER THERAPY FOR COMMON AILMENTS

Ice packs, hot and cold compresses, medicated baths and other forms of water therapy were mainstays of folk medicine for centuries.

Today, high-tech medicine has eclipsed water-based treatments. Yet these treatments—safe, inexpensive and easy to use—remain valuable tools for easing discomfort caused by common ailments...

Medicated baths...

We all know how relaxing a warm bath can be. But not everyone realizes that even greater benefits can be reaped by adding natural ingredients to the water.

•**Apple cider vinegar.** Add a cup to bathwater, and splash a handful over your shoulders, back and chest. That will invigorate you when you're fatigued.

This technique also helps restore the skin's germ-killing natural acidity, which is continually washed away by bathing.

To soothe poison ivy or sunburn, add two cups of vinegar.

•**Bran.** A bran bath eases itching, soothes dermatitis or other skin irritations and eliminates scaly patches.

Sew several handfuls of wheat or oat bran into a cheesecloth pouch. Soak the pouch in hot water for several minutes, then place in a tub filled with tepid water. Squeeze the pouch until the water turns milky.

•**Pine extract.** One capful in a warm bath helps open clogged pores, speeds healing of rashes and relieves muscle fatigue.

Pine extract is available at drugstores and health-food stores. Do *not* confuse it with pine *cleanser*, which will irritate the skin.

Salt massage...

This energizing technique tones tissues, relieves stress and fatigue ...and can help you ward off a cold.

Sit on the edge of a tub filled with warm water. Pour salt into a cupped hand. Slowly add water to the salt until you make a thick paste.

Using firm, circular motions, rub the paste over your body. Then rinse off the paste with a brief soak in the tub...or sponge it off with cold water. Be careful not to rub salt onto sores, cuts, etc.

Hand bath...

To ease writer's cramp, soak hands in hot water. To warm cold hands, soak them alternately in hot water (three minutes) and cold water (30 seconds). Repeat several times, ending with cold water.

Caution: Don't leave hands in cold water for more than a few minutes at a time.

Cold-water treading...

Fill the tub ankle-deep with cold water. Holding onto a firmly anchored rail, march in place for a few seconds or minutes (as long as you can comfortably tolerate). Then rub your feet briskly with a towel.

Done twice daily, this technique creates a remarkable sense of well-being...and is great for relieving exercise-related leg cramps. Some believe that it builds resistance to disease as well.

Done at night, cold-water treading promotes sound sleep—yet it has an eye-opening effect when done in the morning.

Compresses...

To prevent or relieve headache pain, fold a washcloth in half, dip it in ice water and wring it out. Place it on your head or neck. Rewet it every few minutes to keep it cold.

To relieve a sore throat or laryngitis, fold a cotton cloth in thirds, wet it with cold water and wring it out. Wind it once around the neck and fasten with a safety pin. Over the cloth, wrap a wool scarf.

Leave this wrap in place as long as you like. With the cold trapped against the skin by the wool, the body continues to divert more warming blood to the area—helping break up congestion.

Source: Dian Dincin Buchman, PhD, a New York City-based lecturer on water therapy and other alternative therapies. She is the author of several books, including *The Complete Book of Water Therapy*. Keats Publishing.

EXERCISE AND INCONTINENCE

Up to one in three women experiences urine loss while exercising. *Reason:* The muscles responsible for supporting the vagina, bladder and urethra are not strong enough to counteract the increase in abdominal pressure caused by exercise.

Self-defense: Kegel exercises. Contract the anal sphincter as you would to prevent a bowel movement. Hold for a count of four and then relax for a count of four. Perform the exercise continuously for five minutes, repeating twice daily.

Source: Ingrid Nygaard, MD, assistant professor of obstetrics and gynecology, University of Iowa, Iowa City. Her study of 144 female college athletes and 290 other women 17 to 68 years of age was published in *Obstetrics and Gynecology*, 655 Avenue of the Americas, New York 10010.

EXERCISE CURES INSOMNIA

When previously sedentary people followed a four-times-a-week exercise regimen consisting of two 60-minute sessions of aerobics, plus two brisk 30-minute walks, they fell asleep faster and slept longer than they could previously.

Theory: Exercise boosts feelings of well-being, counteracting negative emotions that interfere with sleep.

Source: Abby C. King, PhD, assistant professor of health research & policy and medicine, Center for Research in Disease Prevention, Stanford University, Stanford, CA.

NEW HELP FOR INSOMNIA

A new technology called *low-energy emission therapy* (LEET) promises a safe, drug-free treatment for insomnia—a problem that affects roughly one of every three Americans.

LEET involves exposing the brain to low levels of electromagnetic energy—a much weaker form of the energy released by many electrical appliances.

Preliminary studies in the US and Europe have shown it to be highly effective against chronic insomnia. Other studies suggest that LEET may also be useful for treating certain forms of anxiety and even high blood pressure.

During a LEET session, the patient reclines in bed or in an easy chair with an aluminum "spoon" in his/her mouth. The spoon, connected by wire to an amplifier, delivers the electromagnetic energy. A typical session lasts 20 minutes.

The energy is too weak to be felt by most people—although people with fillings in their front teeth may experience a slight tingle.

LEET does *not* cause immediate sleepiness. Instead, it induces a deep sense of relaxation that makes it easier to sleep later on. People who have tried LEET for several sessions report longer, deeper sleep—and more vivid dreams.

Unlike sleeping pills—which should be taken for no more than a couple of months because of the risk of dependency—LEET can be used safely even for extended periods. If LEET therapy is suddenly discontinued, there is no "rebound" effect. Its effects wear off gradually.

LEET is now being reviewed by the FDA. Approval is expected within two to three years.

Source: Martin Reite, MD, professor of psychiatry, University of Colorado Health Sciences Center, Denver. Dr. Reite has participated in several studies of LEET.

LITTLE-KNOWN APHRODISIACS

Jasmine oil heightens male sexual response by stimulating the region of the brain that controls erections. And it's not the only mood-altering oil. Coriander fights stress and fatigue.

Relaxing: Chamomile, cypress, juniper, marjoram and myrrh. *Stimulating:* Eucalyptus, ginger, pine and rosemary. These "essential oils" can be inhaled from a handkerchief or added to vegetable oils and used in massage.

Source: Jeanne Rose, chairman, National Association of Holistic Aromatherapy, Box 17622, Boulder, CO 80308.

MY LITTLE SECRET FOR CURING A SORE THROAT

A potion made of honey and lemon juice is a well-known—and surprisingly effective—remedy for sore throat. But I've found a way to make it even more potent—simply add cayenne pepper.

Each ingredient serves a purpose. Honey coats the throat, easing irritation and making it easier to talk. Lemon reduces inflammation, while providing lots of virus-killing vitamin C.

The cayenne boosts blood circulation to the area, speeding the natural healing process. Cayenne is also a good source of vitamin A, which is essential for healthy epithelial cells.

This potion can be used instead of cough drops or other sore throat remedies. It is *completely* safe.

Bonus: At seven cents a dose, this potion is cheaper than over-the-counter remedies. They can cost up to $6 for a four-ounce bottle (about 50 cents a dose).

I recommend the honey/lemon juice/cayenne potion whenever any of my patients has a sore throat, cough or even laryngitis. In fact, it's good for almost any upper respiratory tract inflammation.

When my own kids get sore throats, I give them a dose at bedtime. By morning, their symptoms are usually gone.

How to make it: Pour ¾ teaspoon of honey into a tablespoon, then top off the spoon with fresh lemon juice. Add a pinch of cayenne pepper.

The remedy should help you feel better immediately. It may safely be taken up to four times a day.

Source: Elson M. Haas, MD, medical director of the Preventive Medical Center of Marin in San Rafael, CA. He is the author of several books, including *A Diet for All Seasons*. Celestial Arts.

THE CURE-ALL OIL

Every first-aid kit should contain tea tree oil. It helps prevent bacterial and fungal infections *and* acts as a powerful pain-reliever. I use it on bug bites and stings, cuts, scrapes and scratches, ingrown toenails, acne, mouth ulcers and burns.

The oil also can be used on fungal infections, including athlete's foot and jock itch. I even prescribe it in my practice to prevent outbreaks of genital herpes.

Used by aboriginal people in Australia for thousands of years, tea tree oil has been commercially available in this country since the 1920s. It is expected to be approved by the FDA for use as an antiseptic and antifungal.

Use tea tree oil full-strength, right out of the bottle, once or twice daily until the problem clears up. Apply it sparingly with a cotton ball or your fingertip. Or purchase tea tree oil in an applicator bottle with a dropper tip.

Caution: Never drink tea tree oil or put it in your eyes.

To prevent mouth ulcers or genital herpes flare-ups, apply a few drops of the oil at the first sign of an outbreak. If sores are already present, tea tree oil can be used to alleviate discomfort and speed healing.

A good brand of tea tree oil is *Thursday Plantation*. It's available at most health-food stores, or from the manufacturer at 800-848-8966. *Cost:* About $10 for 25 milliliters (about 0.85 ounce). Because you use only a few drops at a time, this isn't costly.

Be sure the bottle specifically states it is oil of *Melaleuca alternifolia*, the botanical name of the tea tree.

Source: Christiane Northrup, MD, an obstetrician–gynecologist practicing in Yarmouth, ME, and assistant clinical professor of obstetrics and gynecology, University of Vermont College of Medicine at Maine Medical Center, Portland. She is the author of *Women's Bodies, Women's Wisdom*. Bantam Books.

AMAZING FLOWER REMEDY HEALS...
AND HEALS...AND HEALS

Dried flowers of *calendula officinalis* are good for burns, cuts, scrapes, acne, tonsillitis and canker sores, vaginitis, rashes, athlete's foot and sunburn.

During the Civil War, these bright orange and yellow flowers provided the major line of defense against infection. Today you can buy dried calendula flowers, ointment, tincture or spray at most health-food stores...or grow your own.

Calendula flourishes in almost any climate, whether it's planted in a pot or in the ground.

Most nurseries sell bedding plants in the springtime. Be sure to ask for *calendula officinalis*—not marigolds.

Flowers harvested between June and September are most potent. Dry them out of direct sun on a mesh screen for one to two weeks. Store in an airtight container.

Hot calendula tea helps soothe ulcers. Gargle with cool tea for inflamed tonsils or canker sores.

To make tea: Pour 10 ounces of boiling water over ⅔ cup of the flowers. Let it steep for 15 minutes. Or add five to 10 drops of calendula tincture to a cup of hot water.

Apply tincture or spray to rashes, cuts, scrapes or acne with a cotton ball. Spraying is good for sunburn, vaginitis and pinworms. Use ointment on scabs, eczema and psoriasis.

To make ointment: Melt ½ cup of petroleum jelly over low heat in a double boiler. Add a handful of dried calendula flowers. Heat on low for an hour. Strain out the herb and pour into a glass jar.

Source: Jamison Starbuck, ND, a naturopathic physician in private practice in Missoula, MT. She is a visiting professor at the National College of Naturopathic Medicine in Portland, OR, and the Southwest College of Naturopathic Medicine in Scottsdale, AZ.

NATURAL STRATEGIES FOR AVOIDING
TROUBLESOME BREAST CYSTS

Breast cancer gets lots of media attention—and rightly so. But far more common is *fibrocystic breast disease.* At some point during their lives, 70% of women develop the fluid-filled, tender or painful breast lumps that characterize this condition.

University of Vermont gynecologist Christiane Northrup, MD, answers the most common questions about breast cysts...

•**What causes breast cysts?** During ovulation and just prior to menstruation, fluctuating hormone levels can cause breast cells to retain fluid—resulting in cysts.

An estrogen/progesterone imbalance also appears to promote cyst development, but doctors don't know exactly how—or why.

In some cases, cysts are linked to abnormally high levels of estrogen. This is usually caused by eating too much fat.

Other women develop breast cysts despite having normal estrogen levels. *Good news:* The lumps usually disappear following menopause.

•**How can I tell a tumor from a cyst?** Cysts typically feel like a bunch of peas or grapes just under the skin. A painful lump is nearly always a cyst. Cancerous lumps are generally not tender.

•**Is breast cancer more common among women who get breast cysts?** In the 1970s, a few studies indicated that this might be the case. But subsequent research at the National Cancer Institute found that the vast majority of fibrocystic breast disease diagnoses did *not* involve an increased risk of cancer.

Exception: About 1% of women with fibrocystic breasts have *ductal atypia*. These abnormal breast cells sometimes turn cancerous.

•**If I discover a lump in my breast, what should I do?** Have your doctor examine it at once. He/she may want to obtain additional tests, such as a mammogram, sonogram or needle aspiration/biopsy.

If the lump contains fluid, odds are it's a cyst. It should disappear once the fluid is removed.

Important: Perform monthly breast self-examinations to spot lumps as early as possible.

•**Are certain women more likely to get breast cysts?** Fibrocystic breasts are more common among women who are sensitive to caffeine…and those who have heavy periods, severe menstrual cramps and/or premenstrual syndrome.

•**The lumps in my breasts are very painful. What can I do for relief?** First, avoid all sources of caffeine. That goes for chocolate and caffeinated soft drinks, as well as coffee and tea. And don't overlook over-the-counter painkillers and diet aids. Many contain caffeine.

To keep your estrogen levels in check, adopt a low-fat, high-fiber diet. This diet should contain no dairy products…and should be high in whole grains, fruits, vegetables and beans. After three months, add dairy foods back into your diet to see if they make a difference.

•**Are nutritional supplements helpful?** Many women get at least partial relief by taking a daily multivitamin or a daily pill containing 400 to 600 international units (IU) of vitamin E.

Also helpful: Selenium (24 to 32 micrograms a day)…vitamin A (1,000 to 5,000 IU a day)…capsules of evening primrose oil, flaxseed oil or black currant seed oil (500 mg four times a day).

•**A friend of mine suggests that I try massage. Is that helpful?** Yes. Massage relieves discomfort by dispersing excess fluid to the lymph glands, where it's channeled out of the body.

What to do: Rub your hands together until they are warm, then massage each breast in concentric circles about 30 times. Use both hands, with your fingertips meeting in the middle. Move clockwise on the right breast, counterclockwise on the left breast.

For persistently painful breast cysts, I often recommend self-treatment with topical iodine. Iodine seems to affect estrogen's ability to bind to breast cells.

Apply iodine tincture in a three-inch-square patch to your upper thigh or lower abdomen. If the stain fades within a few hours, apply it to another area of the upper thigh or lower abdomen.

Repeat these applications as long as they continue to fade within a few hours. When you can see a slight stain that persists for 24 hours, stop the treatment.

Source: Christiane Northrup, MD, assistant clinical professor of obstetrics and gynecology, University of Vermont College of Medicine, at Maine Medical Center, Portland. She is the author of *Women's Bodies, Women's Wisdom.* Bantam Books.

4. Self-Defense

AN UNCONVENTIONAL FAMILY DOCTOR TELLS WHAT PATIENTS DO WRONG

After 44 years as a family doctor, I have come to realize that while doctors are far from perfect...patients make mistakes, too. Here are the most common ones...

Mistake: **Failing to examine your beliefs about illness.** What we think and feel can have a profound effect on our physical health. Doctors have known that for years, yet patients continue to neglect the psychological components of their illnesses.

I have a patient in her mid-50s who was bedridden with back pain for more than three years. As we talked about her situation, she told me she had spent her entire marriage tiptoeing around an overbearing husband.

Gradually she realized that while her back pain was debilitating, it gave her a respite from this unpleasant man.

She also came to realize that he, too, benefited from her incapacity. In playing the devoted caregiver, he became a martyr. He gained the admiration of others in the community.

Once this woman fully understood the link between her pain and her troubled marriage, she told me, *I no longer have to buy into this.* Now she's up and out of bed...and planning on how she will honor her *own* needs. She's even thinking about taking a rafting trip.

I advise all people facing illness to ask themselves, *What can I learn from my illness?* If you take an honest look, you may be surprised to find some answers that will speed the healing process.

Mistake: **Failing to ask questions.** I can't tell you how many times I've had patients gaze at me blankly after I've given a detailed explanation of their condition and outlined a treatment plan.

If you don't understand what your doctor is saying—say so. If he/she suggests a diagnostic test or surgery or prescribes a medication, ask how these will help.

Important: If you're facing a subtle or potentially serious ailment, you need the doctor's undivided attention. Avoid scheduling your appointments for just before noon or at the end of the day. At those times, your doctor may be distracted by thoughts of getting a bite to eat...or going home.

Mistake: **Failing to heed the doctor's advice.** Not too long ago I treated a man with a spastic colon. I prescribed an antispasmodic and asked him to return in a week.

The day before this man's follow-up visit, I happened to stop in at a local drugstore. While there, I saw on a shelf the bottle of medicine with my patient's name. He had given the prescription to the pharmacist but had never returned to get the pills.

At his appointment the next day, the man complained that the pills I had prescribed were no good. When I told him that I knew he had never taken the pills, he said he was sure they wouldn't have helped anyway!

The pharmacist told me that it was common for patients not to pick up their prescriptions.

Mistake: **Expecting immediate results.** Even though diseases can take years to develop and drugs can take days to work, patients generally expect an overnight cure.

Example: Antibiotics are very effective against strep throat. However, they take up to 48 hours before providing any relief—something I always tell my patients. Still, it's not uncommon for a patient or a patient's parent to call me at home the very same evening—and complain that there has been no improvement.

Mistake: **Not being frank with your doctor.** A heart patient I'd been treating for years suddenly got very sick and almost died. Lab tests revealed that he had overdosed on *digoxin.* I had prescribed this drug. At the dose I had ordered for him, however, I couldn't see how he could have overdosed.

It turned out that this man was going to two *other* doctors besides me. Each doctor—myself included—thought that he was the only doctor. Each of us had prescribed *digoxin.*

The man thought that one pill wasn't enough, so he tripled the dose. This faulty reasoning almost cost him his life.

Mistake: **Second-guessing your doctor.** If your doctor suggests a risky operation, it's perfectly sensible to get a second opinion. But don't try to play the role of the doctor when seeking medical care for yourself or a family member.

Example: A friend's octogenarian mother suffered a mini-stroke. After examining her thoroughly, her doctor recommended a series of tests to check for a possible blockage of the carotid arteries in her neck. She declined to have these tests.

Meanwhile, a magazine article convinced her husband that she needed carotid artery surgery. On his advice, this woman traveled to another state and checked into a prestigious clinic.

After several days and a barrage of tests—the same ones recommended by her original doctor—a neurosurgeon at the clinic informed her that the surgery wasn't worth the risk.

This poor woman could have saved lots of time and worry—not to mention much of the clinic's $25,000 fee—simply by letting her doctor perform those tests in the first place.

Mistake: Wasting your doctor's time with silly, insignificant problems. Half of all patients are what I call the "worried well." Each morning, these people wake up, look in their throats, stick out their tongues and feel themselves from head to toe for a lump.

Even the slightest twinge causes these people to rush to the doctor or the emergency room. They're not sick. They *fear* being sick... and want to be assured that they're not.

To minimize the risk of a malpractice lawsuit, doctors who treat such people perform endless tests just to ensure that the twinge isn't the first symptom of a dreaded disease.

Other individuals may have a minor ailment—a cold, a minor skin infection or another insignificant problem. These people don't need a physician. They could treat themselves or simply wait for whatever is bothering them to go away.

Lesson: Learn to trust your own judgment. Wait until you're ill before dashing to the doctor.

This does not mean you should refrain from having regular physical exams. But not every ache requires medical attention. As a result of such foolish behavior, hundreds of millions of dollars are wasted each year on unnecessary medical care.

Source: O.T. Bonnett, MD, a family practitioner in private practice in Raton, NM. He is the author of *Confessions of a Healer: The Truth From an Unconventional Family Doctor.* MacMurray & Beck.

5. Mind Power

BELIEVE IT OR NOT YOUR PERSONALITY TRAITS AFFECT YOUR IMMUNE SYSTEM

After studying mind-body medicine for over 10 years, I've identified seven immunity- boosting emotional traits...

The A.C.E. factor...

A.C.E. stands for "Attend, Connect and Express." Some people are very aware of how they feel physically and emotionally. Others repress their feelings—especially negative ones.

Problem: People who repress feelings miss out on information that can help them stay healthy. Anger, grief, irritation and anxiety are all signs that some aspect of your life is wrong.

Gary Schwartz, PhD, a University of Arizona psychologist, has studied this phenomenon for 20 years. He has found that people who always say that "everything's fine"—even when physical and psychological tests show otherwise—have low levels of disease-fighting white blood cells.

People who admit negative thoughts and feelings have an active immune system...and are less likely than "repressors" to have asthma, rheumatoid arthritis, diabetes or aggressive cancer.

To cultivate the A.C.E. factor in yourself, admit that you may be blocking negative emotions. Don't feel guilty. Just think of repression as a talent that's no longer necessary.

Begin to tune in (attend) to how you're feeling moment by moment. Find a quiet place and sit for a few minutes each day. Be aware of any physical or emotional sensation, including sadness. Try to *connect* these feelings to events in your life.

As your negative feelings come into consciousness, find ways to *express* them. Develop strategies for dealing with the source of those feelings—work, marriage, etc. As you do, you'll begin to restore your emotional balance, and boost your immune system.

The capacity to confide...

James Pennebaker, PhD, a Southern Methodist University psychologist, has taken Dr. Schwartz's work a bit further. He's shown that people who *write* about traumatic events from their past get healthier...and remain healthier.

In Pennebaker's studies, various groups—from students to Holocaust survivors—wrote about painful experiences for 20 minutes a day over four days.

During the six months that followed, they exhibited fewer symptoms of illness. They also went to the doctor less often than a control group who wrote about trivial events.

Subsequent studies confirmed that keeping a journal temporarily boosts the response of key immune system cells called T-lymphocytes. Keeping a journal seems to work if you write about current life events as well. Talking into a tape recorder is not quite as effective as writing.

Consider keeping your own emotional journal. Spend 20 minutes on each session, for at least four days in a row. On the first two days, you may feel worse as painful memories resurface. By day four, pain gives way to understanding and a peaceful sense of resolution.

Write about any issue or feeling that seems relevant. You may or may not choose to show what you've written to others. What really matters is simply confiding in yourself.

Commitment, control and challenge...

This concept was developed by psychologist Suzanne Ouellette, PhD, now at the City University of New York. She hit upon the idea while studying AT&T executives in the late 1970s, when that company was breaking up.

Ouellette noticed that some workers tended to get sick under the stressful conditions, while others remained healthy. Closer study revealed that the "hardy" workers shared three key characteristics...

•**Strong commitment to work, relationships and other pursuits**—including a sense of purpose in what they were doing.

•**Sense of control.** While they might not have controlled everything, they always felt there was *something* they could do to improve the situation.

•**Acceptance of change.** They saw change as a part of life—and acknowledged that it could be positive.

Executives who shared these hardiness traits were half as likely to get sick as those who lacked them.

Ouellette and a colleague have developed a four-part program for increasing hardiness…

•**Find a comfortable place to sit.** Focus on your reaction to a recent stressful event. Look for a word, phrase or image that describes your feelings. You might say simply that you felt bad, for example, or that you felt like a boat on choppy water.

•**Jot down three ways the stressful event could have been worse, and three ways it could have been better.** Explore the different scenarios in your mind.

•**Develop a plan to improve the stressful situation.** This plan should involve gathering other viewpoints and expressing your needs to others.

•**Accept the aspects of the situation you can't change.** Find a way to compensate for your lack of control via a different attitude or approach to the problem.

Assertiveness…

George F. Solomon, MD, a Stanford University psychiatrist and a pioneer in mind-body research, has done several studies linking assertiveness to stronger immunity.

In one study, Solomon examined a group of HIV-positive individuals who had stayed healthy for at least 18 months despite having low T-cell counts. All were highly assertive.

In another study, Solomon studied 20 pairs of sisters in which one of the pair had rheumatoid arthritis. He found that the arthritis-free sisters were far more assertive than their siblings.

To help them boost their assertiveness, Solomon gives his patients permission to attend to their needs. He suggests that they consider pursuing treatments to help them get in touch with these needs, including massage, meditation, psychotherapy and assertiveness training.

Solomon also suggests learning to say "no" when asked to do something you don't want to do—and not being afraid to make requests of others. This may seem selfish, but it's really an acknowledgment of your own needs. In the long run, it will lead to more nourishing relationships.

Affiliative trust…

David McClelland, PhD, a Boston University psychologist, has shown that one measure of our capacity to heal is our ability to bond with others. Those who can trust others have increased resistance to disease.

McClelland tested people using picture stories (ambiguous drawings that reveal unconscious desires and motivations). He found that those who had a need for power—but who had suppressed this need—had lower-than-normal antibody and natural killer cell counts. People who had a strong need for social connections had stronger immunity.

McClelland has identified a health-promoting quality that he calls *affiliative trust*. That's the desire for positive, loving relationships based on mutual respect and trust. Healing damaged relationships is a key element.

Altruism...

Altruism takes affiliative trust to the next level—in which you bond not just with loved ones, but with strangers.

Phyllis Moen, PhD, of Cornell University, followed 420 housewives for 30 years. She found that those who did volunteer work had fewer illnesses and lived longer.

In a recent survey of more than 3,000 volunteers, Allan Luks, executive director of Big Brothers/Big Sisters of New York City, found that people who do volunteer work have better-than-normal health in several different categories.

Self-complexity...

Your ability to live out the many different sides of your personality is linked to strong immunity. Patricia Linville, PhD, a Duke University psychologist, calls this "self-complexity."

People with self-complexity avoid putting all their emotional eggs in one basket. This affords increased protection against life's stresses.

Linville devised a test for self-complexity and tried it on 100 students. *What she found:* Students who rated high in self-complexity were less vulnerable to illness or depression when highly stressed.

To test your self-complexity: Take a piece of paper and mark off columns for various parts of your "self," including different roles, activities, relationships and "sub-personalities." Be sure to include aspects of yourself that you feel have been neglected. Under each column, list personal qualities you exhibit with respect to each self-aspect.

Think about how you can cultivate the aspects of yourself that you've been neglecting. Close your eyes and conjure up an image symbolizing a neglected part of yourself. Ask this image what it wants and needs.

Source: Henry Dreher, a medical writer specializing in mind-body medicine. He is the author of *The Immune Power Personality: 7 Traits You Can Develop to Stay Healthy.* Dutton.

THE JOY OF STRESS

In a recent study of 1,300 heart patients, individuals who did high-stress work were no more likely to suffer a heart attack than individuals with low-stress jobs. Patients with heart disease may *benefit* from stressful work.

Theory: Work gives people a sense of accomplishment and strong social support.

Source: Redford B. Williams, MD, professor of psychiatry, Duke University Medical Center, Durham, NC.

NEW DISEASE FIGHTER: HONESTY

Revealing your true feelings lowers your risk for cancer and heart disease. Dishonesty seems to weaken the immune system, raising the risk of infectious disease.

Helpful: Before responding to any question, ask yourself, *Is what I am about to say truthful?...Is it necessary?...*and *Is it kind?* By reflecting on these three questions, you'll be honest, while not hurting others.

Source: Brad Blanton, PhD, a psychologist in private practice in Washington, DC, and the author of *Radical Honesty.* Dell Trade Paperbacks.

THE FAITH FACTOR

When I wrote *The Relaxation Response* 20 years ago, Americans were just beginning to recognize the physical and mental toll taken on our bodies by psychological stress.

Psychological stress causes the body to pump out adrenaline and other hormones that raise blood pressure, tighten muscles and cause anxiety.

In the book, I described a simple 10-minute exercise—the Relaxation Response—that defuses stress without drugs, equipment or metaphysical mumbo jumbo.

What seemed like a revolutionary breakthrough at the time was actually as old as prayer. In fact, I "discovered" the Relaxation Response during my study of the stress-reducing effects of devotional practices.

From prayer to transcendental meditation, devotional practices share two basic characteristics...

•Repetition of a word, sound, phrase or muscular activity.

•Passive disregard of intrusive thoughts.

My research showed that any activity that included both components triggered the exact *opposite* of the stress reaction.

The Relaxation Response alters production of stress-producing hormones, lowering blood pressure, loosening tense muscles and helping to promote a sense of calm.

Surprisingly, it provides significant benefits for hours *after* you stop eliciting it.

Invoke the Relaxation Response regularly, and your body will become less sensitive to stress *all day long.*

Spiritual stress relief...

In recent years, research has amplified the importance of this basic discovery.

We now know that 60% to 90% of doctor visits are for stress-related ills, including high blood pressure, headache, back pain and insomnia. We have also seen how stress promotes heart disease and exacerbates chronic pain.

In our clinics, thousands of people have improved their health using the Relaxation Response, along with good nutrition and exercise. But we've also hit upon another natural way that mind and body work together for health. I call it the "faith factor."

Research has shown with increasing clarity that the simple act of *believing* something will make you well produces beneficial changes in the body.

It's why patients who "believe" in their doctors are more likely to get well than skeptical patients.

What the studies say...

Last December, the Mind/Body Medical Institute at Boston's Deaconess Hospital hosted a conference that brought together researchers who have been studying spirituality and health. These scientists presented a number of exciting findings...

•In a study of 2,679 people, those who regularly attended religious services were less likely to suffer anxiety, depression and other psychological problems.

•In a study of 232 elderly people who underwent open heart surgery, those who claimed to derive strength and comfort from religion were more likely to be alive six months later.

•Eight separate studies found that religious individuals significantly outlived their nonreligious peers.

The new stress prescription...

Though becoming more spiritual seems to confer many health benefits, I remain convinced that an important tool for maintaining optimum health—and the most potent antidote to stress—is the Relaxation Response.

I urge you to practice the following exercise for 10 to 20 minutes, preferably twice a day...

•**Sit comfortably with your eyes closed.** Relax your muscles, starting with those in your feet and progressing upward. Stretch and relax your arms and hands. Roll your head gently from side to side. Shrug and relax your shoulders.

•**Become aware of your breath as you inhale and exhale naturally.** Each time you breathe out, silently repeat the same word or phrase. A neutral word like "one" works fine. But to activate the faith factor, you should choose a word or short phrase that reflects your personal beliefs.

Christian: The phrase could be, "Our Father, who art in heaven," or "I am the way, the truth and the life."

Jewish: You might say "Shalom" (peace), or "The shield of our salvation," or recite a line from a psalm.

Moslem: Perhaps "Allah."

What if you aren't religious? Pick a word or phrase that represents something you *do* believe in—perhaps "peace" or "love."

•**Think only of the repetitive phrase.** When thoughts or worries intrude, simply let them go. Return to your chosen focus. Don't worry about these lapses…and don't criticize yourself.

Maintain a passive, nonjudgmental attitude. Don't keep asking, "Am I doing it right?" or "Is it working?" Just let it happen. And don't *try* to relax. Simply allow the natural response to take over.

Formal religion and beyond…

If you belong to a church, synagogue or another religious institution, make it a point to attend services. *Also:* Participate in the social activities built around your religion. The sense of belonging and community can be a source of strength and healing.

If you're not formally religious, try to get in touch with *your* sense of the spiritual. You may find that as you start performing the Relaxation Response, you feel the presence of a power, force or energy beyond yourself.

But you don't even have to feel spiritual to mobilize the faith factor. Ask yourself, "What do I believe in?" The human spirit? The brotherhood of man? The power of nature? Love of your family? A healthy, active lifestyle?

Whatever your beliefs, find ways to bring them to life. For some people, it could be an early morning run through the park. For others, it might be volunteering in a homeless shelter.

Source: Herbert Benson, MD, president of the Mind/Body Medical Institute of Deaconess Hospital and Harvard Medical School, and associate professor of medicine at Harvard, both in Boston. A pioneer in the scientific study of mind/body interactions, Dr. Benson is the author of several books, including *Timeless Healing: The Power and Biology of Belief.* Scribner.

HANDS-ON HEALING

Massage and other forms of "bodywork" afford more than a luxurious respite from daily living.

Used on a regular basis, they have a profound effect on overall health and well-being. They're helpful for easing psychological stress *and* for relieving pain and other physical discomfort.

Here are five common health problems and examples of bodywork that offer relief for each…

Muscle tension and soreness…

The most popular technique for relaxing tight, sore muscles is *Swedish massage.*

In this technique, the patient lies on a padded table as the massage therapist, using oil for lubrication, spends 30 to 60 minutes stroking the body with smooth, firmly applied hand movements (gliding, kneading, rubbing, etc.). *Cost:* $30 to $100 a session.

Swedish massage promotes relaxation and pain relief by stimulating the brain's production of "feel-good" compounds called *endorphins*. It also boosts blood flow to the muscles.

Swedish massage also seems to boost the immune system. In one recent study, HIV-positive men who got regular massages had increased levels of natural-killer cells.

Resource: American Massage Therapy Association (847-864-0123).

Another technique that may help chronic muscular problems (including a sore back) is *rolfing*. As in Swedish massage, the patient lies on a padded table. The rolfer uses deep hand pressure to release long-held tension and to literally restructure the *myofascia*. That's the web of connective tissue that links the entire body.

A full rolfing program consists of 10 sessions spaced a week or two apart. Each 60- to 90-minute session focuses on a specific area of the body. *Cost:* $75 to $125 a session.

People who finish the program often report feeling not only more relaxed, but also taller and lighter. The release of deep muscle tension also leads to a heightened sense of mental well-being.

Resource: The Rolf Institute (800-530-8875).

A milder and less invasive approach to relieving deep muscle tension is *myofascial release*. In this technique, the therapist uses slow, gentle stretching motions (without oil) to warm and release the myofascia. The therapist typically feels for the part of the body that's tightest, and works on that area first, applying sustained, light pressure.

Myofascial release can provide effective long-term relief from chronic pain and tight muscles—especially in the neck and shoulders. Patients begin with an initial evaluation, usually followed by two or three sessions. *Cost:* $30 to $100 per hour.

Resource: MFR Treatment Center (800-327-2425).

Soft-tissue injury...

A variant of Swedish massage called *medical massage* is ideal for treating tennis elbow, bursitis, sciatica, sprains and spinal curvature (scoliosis), as well as everyday muscle injuries.

A medical massage session is shorter and more focused than a full-body Swedish massage. The therapist concentrates on the problem area—to boost circulation to the injury and break up scar tissue.

Doctors often prescribe medical massage. To find a medical massage therapist on your own, contact the American Massage Therapy Association.

Back pain...

While medical massage can provide temporary relief from lower back pain, long-term relief is often reported with the *Alexander Technique*.

This form of bodywork—a favorite of dancers and other performing artists—involves a mix of "table work," in which the therapist facilitates better alignment of the client's body and spine, and movement exercises done while sitting and standing.

The goal is to learn a new awareness of how you carry your head, neck and torso.

While you may feel better after a single session, 20 to 30 sessions are typically recommended to fully "internalize" this new way of carrying yourself. *Cost:* $35 to $80 a session.

Resource: North American Society of Teachers of the Alexander Technique (800-473-0620).

Headaches and jaw pain...

Almost any form of bodywork can help sufferers of stress-related headaches feel better. *Craniosacral therapy* works specifically with the head. It is often used to treat temporomandibular joint (TMJ) pain and chronic headaches (including migraines).

In this relatively new technique, the therapist uses *extremely* light pressure to manipulate the bones and soft tissue of the spine and skull.

In addition to headaches and TMJ pain, craniosacral therapy is effective against sinus problems, dizziness, ringing in the ears and even chronic back pain. It's often used on children suffering from paralysis, cerebral palsy, attention-deficit hyperactivity disorder and learning disabilities.

Resource: The Upledger Institute (561-622-4334).

Psychological stress...

When it comes to boosting general health and well-being—both physical and mental—many people swear by the centuries-old Japanese system of massage known as *shiatsu* (also known as acupressure).

A shiatsu therapist uses finger pressure on specific areas of the body associated with the flow of "life energy," known in Japan as *Ki* (pronounced *key*). By balancing this energy, shiatsu practitioners promote blood and lymph circulation and induce a deep sense of relaxation.

Resource: Ohashi Institute (800-810-4190) or the American Oriental Bodywork Therapy Association (609-782-1616).

There are some conditions for which bodywork is inappropriate, or for which special care should be exercised.

If you have a particular medical concern, check with your doctor before starting a bodywork program.

Source: Thomas Claire, the author of *Bodywork: What Type of Massage to Get—and How to Make the Most of It.* William Morrow. A licensed massage therapist, Claire lives, teaches and practices bodywork in New York City.

BEAT STRESS AND DEPRESSION
THE NATURAL WAY

The stress of modern life has given rise to a worldwide epidemic of depression. Mood disorders are more prevalent now than ever before, and they're occurring at younger ages.

What's causing this epidemic? Much of the blame may well rest with technology, and the sweeping lifestyle changes it has encouraged.

Our bodies and brains evolved for a Stone Age existence, when daily life was governed by the rising and setting of the sun and the changing of the seasons. Today, people seem to live at a breakneck pace, 24 hours a day, all year long.

Problem: Fast-paced living brings reduced levels of the neurotransmitter *serotonin*, a key buffer against depression.

On the advice of their doctors, many people have turned to antidepressants to relieve their malaise. For serious depression, that's prudent. However, it often makes more sense to find natural, non-drug ways to boost serotonin levels...

Get more light...

Exposure to bright light has been shown to raise serotonin levels. Unfortunately, indoor lighting averages only 200 to 500 lux. That's too weak to do the trick. Outdoors, sunlight can climb above 100,000 lux.

Being exposed to artificial light *at night* (when our ancestors would have been asleep) throws off the production cycle of *melatonin*. This key neurochemical affects a variety of bodily functions, including serotonin synthesis, making it another important buffer against depression.

Antidote: Get outdoors as much as possible during the day. If you live in a "gray" climate, consider buying a light box (10,000 lux). This device—available for $200 to $400—can be used while reading, exercising or watching TV.

Caution: Light boxes should not be used by people with retinal disease.

Best brands: Apollo Light Systems (800-545-9667), Hughes Lighting Technologies (800-544-4825) and The SunBox Company (800-548-3968).

Also helpful: Dawn simulators. These devices (such as those made by Pi Square, 800-786-3296) use light to awaken you naturally on dark winter mornings.

Seek out negative ions...

Air with high concentrations of negative ions—molecules with an extra electron—is clearly linked to positive moods. Unfortunately, city air contains 10 times fewer negative ions than air in the country or by the seashore. Ion concentrations are even lower inside air-conditioned offices.

Antidote: If you can't live in the country or near the ocean, buy a negative-ion generator. These devices boost serotonin levels, improving mood and promoting sleep.

Be sure the machine you buy generates *small* negative ions. That's the kind shown to yield psychological benefits.

Best brands: Sphere One (201-942-9772) and Bionic Products of America (800-634-4667).

Get more sleep...

Adults today get 20% less sleep than before the invention of the electric light. Most of us need *at least* eight hours of sleep a night. Nearly 50% of Americans get less.

Sleep deprivation produces a sharp decrease in serotonin levels. It is strongly linked to depression.

Antidote: Make sleep a priority. If you feel sleepy during the day, or if you need an alarm clock to wake up, you probably need more shut-eye.

Strategies: Keep the bedroom cool and dark...avoid work or stimulating TV for at least one hour before bedtime...cut down on caffeine and alcohol...exercise late in the day (but at least five hours before bedtime)...rise at the same time each day. On days when you can't get the sleep you need, nap.

Get regular exercise...

Exercise—an excellent serotonin booster—is linked not only with better moods, but also with better overall health. Yet despite the so-called "fitness revolution," Americans get less exercise today than even 10 years ago. We get *far* less exercise than our hunter-gatherer ancestors.

Antidote: Find an exercise you enjoy, and do it regularly. Aerobic exercise several times a week is ideal, but *any* kind of exercise is better than none.

Rethink your diet...

Our ancestors survived mostly on green plants and small game animals, which were low in fat but *high* in cholesterol. *Lesson:* While some middle-aged men and others at high risk for heart attack should take steps to lower high cholesterol levels, cholesterol levels below 160 confer a heightened risk of depression, accidents and suicide. Apparently, low cholesterol levels interfere with the regulation of serotonin.

That doesn't mean we should binge on saturated fat. It does suggest that we should be wary of cholesterol levels that are too high *or* too low.

What about carbohydrates? They do appear to improve serotonin function *temporarily*. Over the long term, however, a high-carbohydrate diet diminishes your sense of well-being.

Reason: Carbohydrates quickly raise blood sugar and insulin levels. Elevated insulin signals the body to store food as fat—making it less available for energy. Insulin also boosts production of certain prostaglandins linked to depression.

Antidote: Eat a diet that's more in line with that of our hunter-gatherer ancestors...

•**Emphasize fruits and vegetables while limiting consumption of grains and sweets.** When you do eat grain, stick to whole grains. They have a less drastic effect on blood sugar than white bread or processed cereal.

•**At every meal, maintain a protein-fat-carbohydrate calorie ratio of 30%–30%–40%.**

•**Keep meals under 500 calories.** Don't let more than five hours pass between meals (except when you're asleep). Frequent, small meals keep insulin levels lower than a few large meals.

•**Do not eat red meat or egg yolks more than once a week.** These foods contain a chemical precursor to a brain chemical that is associated with depression.

What about antidepressants?

Anyone who is so depressed that he/she has trouble functioning at work or at home should seek a medical diagnosis.

Fluoxetine (Prozac) is the best known of a group of antidepressants called *selective serotonin re-uptake inhibitors* (SSRIs). These drugs avoid many of the serious medical risks of older drugs. But Prozac can cause decreased libido, delayed orgasm, insomnia and agitation...and may suppress melatonin levels.

Over the short term, this is probably not a concern. For patients who take the drug for a year or more, however, the effect on melatonin might have negative implications for long-term mood and health.

Sertraline (Zoloft) and *paroxetine* (Paxil) are similar to Prozac but may be better or worse in a given individual.

Fluvoxamine (Luvox) is another SSRI that appears to have fewer side effects than Prozac. Unlike Prozac, it *raises* melatonin levels.

Nefazodone (Serzone)—the newest antidepressant on the US market—affects serotonin more subtly and seems free of Prozac's most objectionable side effects. It may be particularly helpful in treating depression accompanied by anxiety or insomnia.

Venlafaxine (Effexor) acts on serotonin and boosts levels of *norepinephrine* (the neurochemical affected by earlier antidepressants called *tricyclics*). It has a good track record in treating cases that fail to respond to other medication.

Bupropion (Wellbutrin) does not act on serotonin. In fact, we're not quite sure *how* it works. In a tiny percentage of cases, it has been associated with seizures. This risk can be minimized by lowering the dosage and spreading doses out throughout the day.

Source: Michael J. Norden, MD, clinical associate professor of psychiatry at the University of Washington, Seattle. He was among the first to publish medical accounts of the varied uses of Prozac and has been a pioneer in the integration of psychopharmacology and alternative treatments. Dr. Norden is the author of *Beyond Prozac*. ReganBooks/HarperCollins.

THE MARDUS MANEUVER

Remember the last time a friend urged you to "relax" when you were feeling upset?

That counsel probably wasn't too helpful. When you're truly worried or anxious, it's simply *impossible* to make yourself feel relaxed.

Nervousness arises from the "fight or flight" response built into the body's autonomic nervous system (ANS). The ANS cannot be turned on or off by an act of will.

It turns on automatically when it senses danger—a sudden noise, an angry voice or even a troubling thought. It floods the bloodstream with adrenaline, causing your palms to sweat, your heart to race and your muscles to tense. Try to "calm" this adrenaline, and you'll only become frustrated and upset.

Relaxation techniques like deep breathing, meditation and yoga can help *prevent* anxiety. But these techniques are of little use if you're *already* anxious. In fact, they tend to produce the opposite effect—much like a friend who urges you to relax.

Many therapists persist in using relaxation techniques as a primary treatment for anxiety. In my work as a stress-management counselor, however, I've had better success with a different approach.

Instead of having my clients try to "relax" their worries away, I teach them to turn anxiety into excitement—in other words, to turn "bad" anxiety into "good."

Making worry work for you...

A worry is a negative thought about something over which you have no control. You're releasing adrenaline not over a real threat, but over an imagined one.

There's nothing you can do with this adrenaline. You can fight an attacking dog, but you can't fight or resolve a fear. As a result, you feel stuck, tense and unhappy.

A few years ago, I discovered a simple technique for turning worry into excitement. My inspiration came from an unlikely place —skydivers.

The moment before leaping from the plane, first-time skydivers are terrified. Once the parachute opens, however, this intense fear turns instantly into exhilaration. What happens? Their terror is channeled into a feeling of incredible "aliveness."

You can apply this scenario to your own fears. Replace your fearful, out-of-control fantasy (worry) with an exciting fantasy that gives you a feeling of personal control.

The Mardus maneuver...

With a little practice, a technique that I call the Mardus maneuver can provide relief from worry in just one second.

What to do: Whenever a worry arises, think instead of something exciting—a sexual encounter, winning the lottery, acing a tennis serve at the US Open, etc.

I call these positive fantasies "the new R & R." That's because they tend to be *risqué* or physically *risky*.

To test the physiological benefits of the Mardus maneuver, I've tried monitoring my clients with biofeedback equipment.

What I've found: Each client registers a rise in adrenaline when I ask him/her to worry. When he/she switches to an exciting fantasy, there's an even higher surge of adrenaline. But the client has a smile ...and reports feeling not anxious, but good. Like the opening parachute, the exciting fantasy turns bad stress into good stress.

The best part of this technique is that the "good" stress is closely followed by a natural and automatic feeling of relaxation.

This technique can be used any time a worrisome thought pops up. It can also be applied to specific problem areas of your life.

Overcoming insomnia...

What makes insomnia so unbearable is not only the loss of sleep, but also the constant *worrying* associated with sleeplessness.

If you're suffering from insomnia, try to convert the worry of "bad" insomnia into "good" insomnia. *What to do:* As you lie in bed, conjure up a "risqué or risky" fantasy.

Apply that same feeling to your present situation. From good insomnia, you'll pass into a state of relaxation. You may even drift off to sleep. If a phantom fear pops back up, just dive back into your "R & R," and repeat the process.

Burning out a worry...

Another way to gain control over your ANS is to worry *on purpose*. My work with biofeedback has shown that a worry always precedes a rush of adrenaline—which makes you feel more worried. In other words, although worries may seem to just happen to us, we actually *make* them happen.

Here's how to break this cycle. Imagine you're at an old-fashioned drive-in movie theater. Project your worry on the big screen for 20 seconds or so. Show the worry in full color, in all its fearsomeness.

Next, imagine one of those refreshment-stand commercials, with talking hot dogs and dancing soda cups. Enjoy this ad for 20 seconds, then go back to your worry movie for another 20 seconds. Continue this for a few cycles, and you'll notice that you're no longer taking your worry movie very seriously.

Procrastination...

Any unpleasant or difficult task is made many times worse by the self-imposed anxiety of procrastination.

The logic of procrastination is, *I can't do this now, because I don't have the time* (or the resources, or the energy, etc.).

Like fear, procrastination causes the release of adrenaline, which makes you enervated and anxious. *Instead:* Move from the "thinking" stage to the "doing" stage.

Example: Procrastinating about cleaning your house? Instead of fretting, take control of your situation by entering the *doing* stage. Pick up one piece of clothing *right now.*

Follow the five-minute rule. For the next five minutes, vow to automatically do whatever you've been worrying about. Do not stop to think. After five minutes, take a break. Ask yourself, *Do I want to continue the task?* If so, continue working. Even if the answer is "no," you've managed to assert control.

This new-found control will make you feel better and in charge... and it will move you a step closer to completing your task.

Dealing with anger...

Some people deal with anger by bottling it up inside. I call these people "stuffers." Others let anger out by yelling at someone or something. I call them "yellers."

Problem: Neither approach can meet your four basic needs when you're angry. These needs are...

•To feel better.

•To remain "connected" to the person who upset you.

•To get an apology for, or an explanation of what hurt you.

•To avoid feeling guilty when expressing your anger.

Stuffing your anger makes you feel worse because it involves withdrawing from the source of your anger. By not speaking up, stuffers ensure that they will not get an apology or acknowledgment.

Yellers suffer, too. They pretend to be in control but really aren't. And by pushing others away, they cut off communication. Of course, once they cool off, they feel guilty for having blown up.

There's another option. By expressing your anger in a clear, first-person statement, you gain control over your angry feelings...and meet these four goals. You're not fighting your upset feelings but learning to channel them instead.

Imagine stubbing your toe on a box on your way to an important meeting. If you tend to stuff your anger, you'll probably hold your breath, wince and pretend it didn't hurt. If you're a yeller, you might curse, or rant against whoever put the box there in the first place.

Better: Say something like, *Ow, I just banged my toe, and I'm really hurting.*

By following this third approach, you...

...feel better physically, because you're asserting control over your situation.

...deal directly with the source of your anger.

...avoid feeling guilty.

...are more likely to get help and understanding from others—perhaps even an apology from whoever left the box there.

The world is full of stresses, and you'll never eliminate all of them. But you'll be happier and more relaxed if you realize that instead of fighting your own negative feelings, you can learn to control them.

The ANS works automatically, but the system has two buttons—one marked "worry," the other marked "excitement." By learning to press the excitement button when you're stressed, you begin to control your phantom fears.

Source: Craig B. Mardus, PhD, a stress-management consultant based in Williamstown, MA, and a consultant to the Canyon Ranch Spa in Lenox, MA. He is the author of *How to Make Worry Work for You: Simple and Practical Lessons on How to Be Happy.* Warner Books.

JOURNAL WRITING CAN BOOST HEALTH

Diaries and journals preserve meaningful experiences, tell life stories and reveal the writer's unique traits and qualities. Writing about feelings can boost the immune system, favorably affect blood pressure and heart rate, and help people cope with pain. Writing is especially helpful for people who have difficulty sharing feelings with others. Explore your deepest emotions and thoughts.

Helpful: Set aside 20 minutes on three or four consecutive days. Write for the full time, without regard to grammar, spelling, punctuation or style.

Source: James Pennebaker, PhD, professor of psychology, Southern Methodist University, Box 750442, Dallas 75275.

HUMOR HELPS KEEP YOU WELL

A sense of humor improves the sense of well-being. *To add humor to your life:* Look for absurd, silly activities around you. Take a humor break every day to read jokes, listen to a funny tape or play with a small child.

Source: Joel Goodman, EdD, director, The Humor Project, 110 Spring St., Saratoga Springs, NY 12866.